YOGA FOR KIDS AND THEIR GROWN-UPS

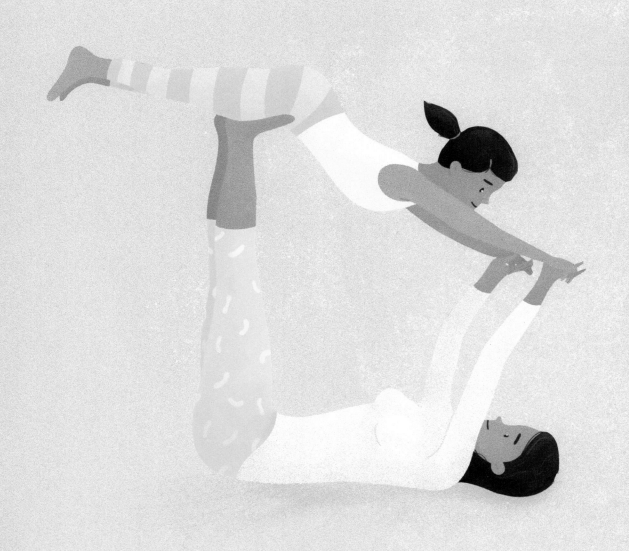

Yoga for Kids

and Their Grown-Ups

100+ FUN YOGA AND MINDFULNESS ACTIVITIES TO PRACTICE TOGETHER

Katherine Priore Ghannam

ILLUSTRATIONS BY TANYA EMELYANOVA

ROCKRIDGE PRESS

For Olive and Zahra,
my light and joy.
To Riyad, for the comic relief
and cosmic support in this great
parenting adventure.

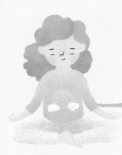

Contents

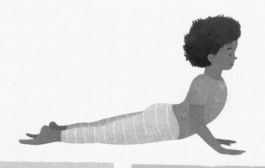

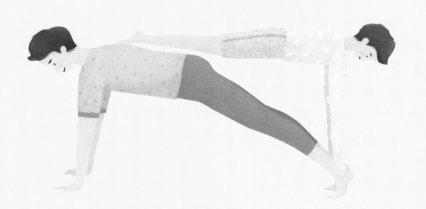

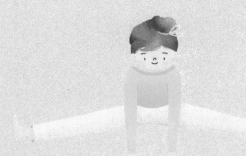

INTRODUCTION

Imagine 33 quiet and serene nine-year olds (with a few wiggles here and there) resting their bodies and taking deep breaths together in the middle of a busy school day. When asked to describe how they feel afterward, one child waves his hand furiously and proudly proclaims, "I feel like a newborn baby!" His classmates nod and wave their hands in agreement. Yoga—a practice of unifying movement with breath and awareness—holds the incredible potential to make us feel new again. For the developing child, this is a powerful and empowering experience.

Yoga and mindfulness provide a source of strength and stability in my work with children, both as an educator and mother to two loving and wildly creative—and just plain wild—toddlers. Not only do these practices relieve stress and encourage a compassionate attitude, they also help children and adults alike slow down and discover their feelings, uncovering their unique assets. We all benefit when we know what makes us tick.

My belief in the power of yoga for children led me to start Headstand, a nonprofit organization that helps integrate yoga and mindfulness programming in K–12 schools. Since its inception in 2008, Headstand has served over 12 thousand students in the San Francisco Bay Area, New York, and Houston. Headstand's program combines yoga, mindfulness practices, and physical activity to teach the skills students need to process feelings, manage stress, develop a sense of self and compassion for others, and support academic achievement. Headstand's online series for K–12 teachers and administrators reaches educators around the globe.

Similar yoga and mindfulness programs for children are flourishing in the United States and abroad. A National Institutes of Health (NIH) study in 2016 found that over 940 schools in the United States alone have implemented a formal yoga program for students. Thousands of classroom teachers are trained to teach mindfulness and yoga to students throughout their day. There are yoga classes and even entire studios that cater to children, integrating games, music, and playful activities. P.E. teachers and coaches often provide yoga and mindfulness routines to improve focus and flexibility.

Yoga encourages children to tap into the vast reservoir of possibility within, which can help them meet their own personal challenges with compassion. Yoga guides children to discover the potential for positive change that exists in all of us.

In a world where we are constantly flooded with information, it's critical to find ways to unplug and connect with our loved ones. As parents and caregivers, we need to provide healthy tools for children to tune out the distractions of everyday life and tune in to their thoughts and feelings. Yoga's physical and emotional benefits for children (and adults!) are profound. These benefits include:

- Holistic mind-body connection
- Self-acceptance
- Increased confidence
- Reduced stress
- Improved concentration and focus

- Increased care for others/empathy
- Decreased negative affect or emotions
- Decreased anxiety in general (and test anxiety in particular)
- Increased sense of calmness and relaxation

Yoga is a way to engage everyone in the family with movement-based play or quiet, calming activities. Yoga provides a simple, easy-to-access, and cost-effective way to help children build physical and emotional awareness. In its most basic form, yoga invites us to pause and take a deep breath, a most valuable tool for parents, caregivers, and children alike.

Yoga and mindfulness routines for kids and parents provide a fun and meaningful way to spend time together at home, in the park, or even on an airplane. Whether you're roaming around the house pretending to be a lion or creating a whole-family partner pose, the yoga activities in this book are sure to engage little ones and deepen family connections.

The book begins with the basics of yoga and mindfulness, providing deeper context for the benefits and a framework for turning these practices into everyday habits. We'll dive into the various types of yoga poses, games, meditations, and relaxation activities, guiding you through different ways to explore yoga with children ages 3 to 12. There are also sample sequences to help you put all the pieces together into a satisfying yoga session.

Explore this book in the way that is most useful to you. You can use it as a guide for poses and a reference for different yoga activities, in which case you might want to jump around. It can also be used as a chronological overview from start to finish. Keep the book on hand as you practice and build routines for yoga and mindfulness with your child or the children in your life.

Most importantly, take a deep breath and dive in with the knowledge that you'll discover pathways for the entire family to connect and play. Now let's get started!

CHAPTER

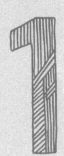

EMPOWERING

KIDS

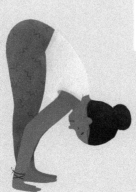

THROUGH

YOGA

Before we get into the specifics of a yoga practice with kids, let's take a closer look at the power of yoga and its unique benefits for children. Yoga builds compassion and self-awareness and can soothe children during challenging times. Yogis of all ages gain a sense of peace and calm, as well as confidence, through the practice of yoga. Once children begin to feel and experience the benefits of yoga, they'll have an inner resource to call on when grown-ups aren't around. Self-soothing is an important skill that will help kids through all stages of life—even deep into adulthood. In short, yoga can play a powerful role in nurturing a kind, confident, and empowered child.

INTRODUCTION TO YOGA

Yoga is an ancient practice of linking physical movements—the yoga poses—with breath and awareness. Originally, yoga was built as a method to encourage the body to sit for longer increments of time during meditation. Holding a pose focuses and calms the mind, and thus is a form of meditation. Today, yoga utilizes yoga sequences—series of poses done in a certain order—for improved physical and mental health. Comprehensive yoga classes emphasize pose sequences, breathing techniques, relaxation, and meditation. There are many types of yoga classes—you can find a yoga class for just about anything, including low-back pain, anxiety, or even laughing! That's right, there are entire classes dedicated to "laughing yoga." A class can be very physical and athletic or relaxing and restorative. A skilled yoga teacher guides students through the poses and meditations with the ultimate goal of building a healthier body and quieter mind.

YOGA PRINCIPLES FOR KIDS AND PARENTS

When starting a yoga practice with kids, there are a few principles that will help make it a rewarding, fun, and nourishing experience.

Tap into Humor! Whenever we attempt to teach children new skills or offer a new experience, a sense of humor can be helpful. Whether it's laughing at ourselves when we fall out of a balancing pose or being a little silly while trying out the cat or dog poses, yoga presents an opportunity to model lightheartedness and fun. It's important to build joy into the everyday rhythms of family life and relationships, and this is a skill we can hone when practicing yoga together. While the benefits are profound, yoga doesn't need to be taken too seriously. It doesn't matter whether you can stand on your head or balance on your arms—anyone can have fun while moving their body into the different poses and bringing awareness to their breath.

Cultivate Compassion and Trust. A compassionate attitude sets the foundation for learning. When you demonstrate kindness and patience with your child, she feels empowered and safe to try new things and will emulate your positive behaviors. Yoga allows our children to experiment and play with new poses and ideas without being graded or judged. At the same time, yoga encourages parents to show children love, support, and acceptance. Yoga exemplifies that we value wellness for our bodies, minds, and hearts.

Get Curious. Encouraging your child's sense of curiosity is important. A curious nature can take us far in both yoga and life. When we approach challenges with openness and curiosity rather than fear, we remain engaged and willing to learn. When you witness your child striving too hard or struggling with a yoga pose, avoid saying "now take a deep breath." Instead, try asking "what happens if you take a deep breath right now?" Or if you start falling out of a yoga pose while practicing with your child, you might say "Wow, that's interesting! I notice I keep falling when I place my foot so high in Tree pose. I think I'll see what happens if I do the other version with my foot on the ground." Using language and action to guide curiosity empowers children to explore and become comfortable in discovering what feels best for them.

Maintain a Growth Mind-set. Carol Dweck, a psychologist and educator at Stanford, is a leading researcher in the education field. Her work demonstrates that a child's belief that she can improve in any area of life, such as schooling, athletics, or friendships, is more important than her innate talent or ability. Dweck makes the case for the long-term benefits of practice and hard work: "The passion for *stretching yourself* and sticking to it, even (or especially) when it's not going well, is the hallmark of the growth mind-set. This is the mind-set that allows people to thrive during some of the most challenging times in their lives." Yoga provides the perfect opportunity to engage in a growth mind-set because it's not about the end goal—it's a practice.

Develop Authentic Communication. When we build yoga routines into our daily lives, they help everyone in the family reduce stress, become more self-aware, and practice empathy. When we are feeling confident, compassionate, and calm, we are able to communicate with more ease, which improves the overall family dynamic. Feeling safe and nurtured helps us express ourselves more clearly and mindfully.

YOGA AND MINDFULNESS

Mindfulness is the ability to pause and become aware of our thoughts in the present moment. According to leading mindfulness expert Jon Kabat-Zinn, "Mindfulness is awareness that arises through paying attention, on purpose, in the present moment, nonjudgmentally . . . It's about knowing what is on your mind."

You can practice mindfulness anytime and anywhere, as it's simply the practice of becoming aware of your thoughts and feelings.

Let's say I'm at the grocery store and there is a long line. When I'm not engaging mindfully (and let's be honest, nobody on the planet is mindful 100 percent of the time), I may end up looking at my phone or even projecting irritation toward the checkout person. But if I have the presence of mind to catch myself in the moment and acknowledge my feelings, I can say to myself "I'm noticing that my heart is beating a bit faster now and I feel agitated and anxious. I have a lot to accomplish today and standing in this line is stressing me out. I'm going to be late to pick up my child from school now." Simply noticing the way we feel takes some of the power out of the emotion and gives us a choice of how to react.

When we become mindful of our feelings, we give ourselves the gift of awareness. In the case above, I can continue to stand in line, indulging my feelings of annoyance or agitation, or I can use the opportunity to take a few deep breaths and practice patience and possibly even compassion. This may enable me to be kind to the grocery checkout person versus snappy or short.

Mindfulness and yoga are intrinsically linked. When practicing yoga, a great deal of mindfulness is required. We are not practicing yoga if we are simply moving our bodies in seemingly strange ways without paying attention to our breath and the thoughts and feelings that arise. The essence of yoga is in bringing awareness to your breath and noticing what's happening in your body and mind.

Mindfulness is a practice that kids can engage in, too. Kids are empowered when they understand their feelings and can begin to make sense of their thoughts. Building the mindfulness muscle creates awareness and builds empathy in our children. As a first step, you can encourage kids to be more mindful simply by modeling mindfulness in your daily life.

The yoga and meditation activities in this book are designed to encourage mindfulness for you, your child, and within your interactions. As the guide for your family, try encouraging mindfulness during yoga in the following ways:

Narrate your own feelings and thoughts:

"Oh, wow! My heart felt so happy when I saw you help your little brother with that pose. How did it feel for you to help him?"

Narrate what you witness:

"Makeyla, you look so focused. I see you taking deep breaths and building that concentration muscle in Tree pose right now."

Encourage compassion and inquiry:

"Whoa. I see you really want to get into this pose. What happens if we go a little slower and just do our best? I love this version of the pose, too." (Modeling a simpler version of the yoga pose.)

As you work through the book, you'll have the opportunity to engage in a more formal mindfulness practice with each pose provided. Cultivating mindfulness while wagging your tail in Down Dog or sitting still in Lotus pose makes it a joyful practice for both parents and kids.

THE BENEFITS FOR KIDS

Yoga combines visualization, mindfulness, and breathing exercises with movement to give children tools to reduce stress and find balance in their minds and hearts. We now know that emotional health is fundamental to academic success, and yoga is a wonderful way to foster the self-care and self-knowledge that help children thrive. Practicing yoga has many incredible benefits for kids of all ages.

BUILDS CONFIDENCE

Yoga has the tremendous power to build confidence in children of all ages, shapes, and abilities. Whether your child is extremely athletic and looking to increase flexibility, or a bookworm with little interest in athletics, yoga provides the opportunity to try new physical challenges in a safe, accepting environment. When children attempt new yoga poses or sit still for minutes at a time, we encourage them to breathe through fear and apprehension, a skill that easily transfers into everyday situations. Overcoming fears on the yoga mat leads to more confidence in approaching challenges in life. When children overcome perceived obstacles, their confidence grows.

REDUCES ANXIETY

Yoga and mindfulness regulate the physiological systems associated with anxiety. According to Harvard Medical School, "By reducing perceived stress and anxiety, yoga appears to modulate stress response systems. This, in turn, decreases physiological arousal—for example, reducing the heart rate, lowering blood pressure, and easing respiration. There is also evidence that yoga practices help increase heart rate variability, an indicator of the body's ability to respond to stress more flexibly." This means yoga can actually help counteract the triggers for anxiety, leading to lower stress levels and more peace of mind in adults and children.

BUILDS FOCUS AND CONCENTRATION

The ability to focus and concentrate in today's information-driven world is a critical skill. A yoga practice requires turning off your phones and screens to spend time focusing on your breath and body. When faced with a physical challenge in yoga, it is almost impossible to dwell on future or past concerns. Yoga encourages us to be in the present moment. As kids practice yoga, they develop the ability to focus on the task or situation at hand, which helps them with school, activities, and general problem solving.

TEACHES SELF-CARE

Learning the art of self-care at an early age builds the foundation for a healthier and happier future. This is an especially powerful aspect of yoga for our kids. Yoga and mindfulness ask our children to understand what it means to take good care of our bodies, minds, and hearts. It builds a practice that is nurturing and, over time, keeps us in better physical and mental health. Time spent doing yoga may be the only time throughout the day in which a child is asked to focus only on herself. Children are empowered when they understand the benefit of a deep breath and how to keep their body physically fit.

YOGA AND ADHD

According to a report from the Centers for Disease Control and Prevention (CDC), approximately 11 percent of children 4 to 17 years of age (6.4 million) have been diagnosed with attention deficit hyperactivity disorder (ADHD). Commonly treated by doctors with medications such as Adderall or Ritalin, many parents and caregivers also seek additional therapies to assist with their child's diagnosis. Yoga and mindfulness are believed to help children with ADHD because the practices can help kids release energy and improve concentration. Yoga practice can be fluid, with a variety of activities, or systematic, with repetition of poses and breathing exercises. Observe what works best for your child and use the activities she's drawn to as building blocks for engagement. As with any activity, your child may demonstrate a range of interest anywhere from extreme dislike to enthusiasm. Some of the students with ADHD I've worked with have discovered the power of yoga and mindfulness only after *years* of resistance. Stick with it and take the little victories—if your child can take smooth and deep breaths for even a minute, she will feel the impact.

PROMOTES SELF-AWARENESS

Yoga and mindfulness teach children introspection, self-regulation, and the self-awareness necessary to respond to challenges instead of hastily reacting to them. One of my former eighth-grade students said after yoga class "I felt so centered, like I really connected with my body and myself." Yoga helps us get to know our inner self, and greet feelings and thoughts that may otherwise go ignored or neglected. This self-awareness helps children in all their interactions.

BUILDS FLEXIBILITY AND BALANCE

You do not have to be able to touch your toes in order to increase flexibility through the practice of yoga. Yoga moves the body in all directions and activates bilateral movement. When you build a practice of forward folds, backbends, side bends, and twists, you increase the body's intelligence, improve flexibility, and create new pathways for creative movement. In fact, according to a study in the *International Journal of Yoga,* after only 10 weeks of yoga, a group of athletes had "significant" gains in flexibility and balance. Another study from the American Council on Exercise revealed even quicker results in flexibility: "After eight weeks, the average flexibility of the yoga group improved by 13 percent to 35 percent and the gains were significantly greater than the non-yoga group."

REWARDS FOR THE FAMILY

Practicing yoga together as a family provides a bonding experience and is a meaningful opportunity for family members to express empathy, show support and encouragement, and learn from each other. Yoga can help strengthen many important aspects of family life.

CONNECTION AND REFLECTION

Because yoga and mindfulness are soothing and nurturing practices, yoga gives each person time and space to connect internally and with one another. The power of even one deep breath can make an impact on our interactions with each other. Yoga is also a time to communicate interest in one another: How are you feeling right now? Is there anything I can do to support you? What do we all hope to get out of this practice? How can we show kindness today? Building reflective questions into your family routine strengthens connection and will have a ripple effect out to your neighbors and community.

GRATITUDE

A sense of appreciation for oneself, each other, and the simple gifts of the world at large can make a big impact on our families and our outlook on life. During yoga, encourage your family to appreciate beauty and comfort as well as the more meaningful aspects of life like all the ways you try to take care of each other. When we express thanks to one another it helps us feel seen and appreciated. Plus, gratitude has been proven to increase both physical and psychological health. According to a 2012 study published in *Personality and Individual Differences*, people with a regular practice of gratitude even feel fewer aches and pains! Gratitude also subdues or eliminates toxic emotions like resentment and anger.

Help children feel a sense of pride and love by expressing your appreciation for them. A simple message goes a long way, such as "Thank you so much for helping me set the table. I feel happy when we work together as a team." Guide children to get in a gratitude habit by starting out yoga time with the question "What are you grateful for today?"

MINDFUL PLAY

Yoga games and activities teach us to play together in ways that also invite mindfulness. It's possible to engage with yoga poses in a distracted and hurried way. But the most important aspect of a strong yoga practice is being mindful. When we are mindful in yoga, it extends to other aspects of our life and gives us more balance through challenges. If you find yourself or your child rushing through your practice or feeling frustrated by the fact that you cannot achieve a certain pose, bring your attention back to your breathing. When we focus on the breath, we coax ourselves into mindfulness. Yoga is not meant to produce additional anxiety. Keep an open mind and attitude as you play together in the poses, always being mindful and having fun!

RELAX AND RENEW

Learning to relax and renew in healthy ways benefits the entire family. Many modern parents feel like there is an endless to-do list and can get so caught up in busyness that they miss opportunities to relax. The yoga relaxation activities and meditations in this book require us to slow down and nourish ourselves without any screens or distractions. There are few activities that allow us to relax together while simultaneously gaining physical and mental health benefits. Watching a movie together is fun and relaxing but does not produce the same health benefits as yoga. A practice of relaxation also teaches kids the value and benefit of self-care. When we are relaxed, we can connect with each other in more meaningful and productive ways.

YOGA AND AUTISM

Children with autism spectrum disorder have individual needs, and only you know your child's preferences and limits. Yoga can assist your child in feeling more connected to his body and in soothing and calming the nervous system. Yoga can also be effective in terms of improving social and communication skills. One study indicated that yoga may "offer benefits as an effective tool to increase imitation, cognitive skills and social-communicative behaviors in children with ASD." In addition, children exhibited increased skills in eye contact, sitting tolerance, nonverbal communication and receptive communication skills (Radhakrishna, S., 2010).

Try using one or two simple, set sequences or routines with your child first. This removes the element of surprise and might feel soothing and systematic to the nervous system. Frequent use of yoga poses can provide physical benefits as you build balance and motor skills with your child. Create a calming environment by dimming the lights, providing props that might assist with sensory stimulation, like a soft and heavy eye pillow or pleasant music. Over time, yoga poses and breathing exercises might be used when emotions begin to escalate. Use the practices in this book as a guide and trust your own experience and knowledge with the individual needs of your child as you integrate yoga and mindfulness into your routines.

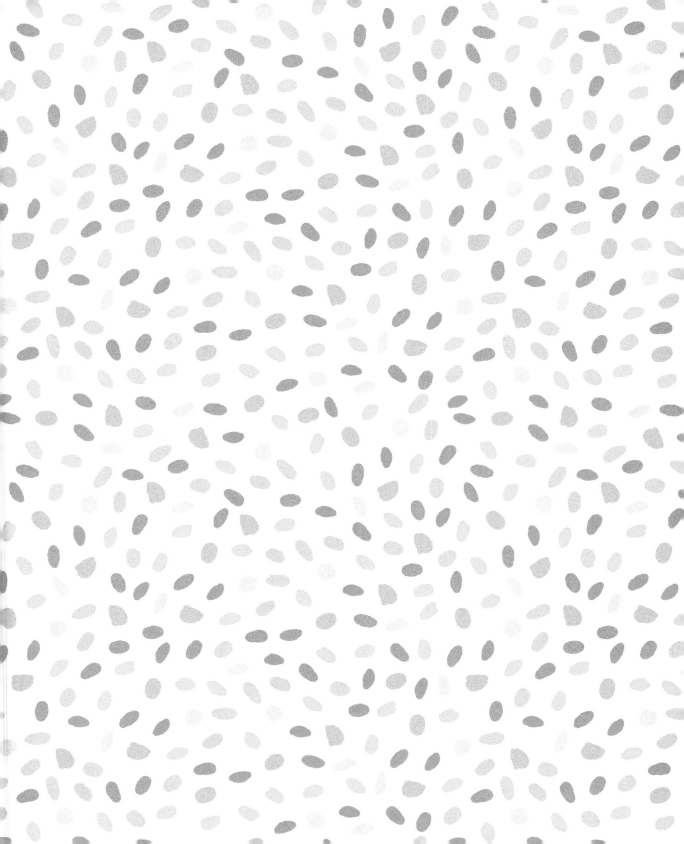

CHAPTER

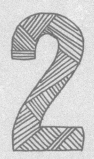

2

FAMILY
YOGA
TIME

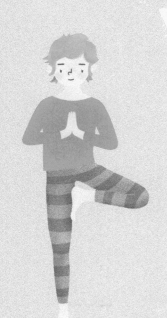

Now it's time to start planning your family yoga time! Before we get into the specific poses and sequences, there are some things to keep in mind as you build out your yoga sessions. Yoga time with kids needs to offer a lot of variety—otherwise little ones can quickly lose interest. That's why I've included lots of options for the various building blocks of a dynamic yoga practice. You'll learn how to mix and match so your sessions best suit the needs of your family. Many of the yoga activities energize and build strength while simultaneously calming the nervous system. Other activities are designed for relaxation and stillness through visualization, breathing, or meditation. Get ready to breathe, move, play, and relax in your home or on the go as you make yoga a regular family activity.

BUILDING BLOCKS

The building blocks of yoga include breathing, meditation, yoga poses, sequences, games, and relaxation. This book offers exercises and activities for each building block. You'll find that some people are drawn to a slow, deeply therapeutic practice of yoga and others enjoy a more active or athletic practice. Take the time to figure out which approach best suits your family on any given day. Whether you are a beginner or an advanced practitioner, the building blocks of yoga will help you generate creative, restorative, and fun yoga sessions for adults and kids.

BREATH

Building a connection to your breath is the foundational practice of yoga—otherwise you are simply moving your body around into funny shapes! Yoga helps us build a habit of attention to the breath. Many yoga traditions suggest breathing in and out through the nose. This is not always appropriate for kids (especially younger toddlers), but simply growing attuned to the breath and noticing it flow in and out during practice is enough to feel the benefits. Chapter 3 (page 27) features 10 breathing exercises you can try with your kids.

POSES

Yoga poses allow us to be active in a way that builds strength, flexibility, and concentration and soothes the nervous system. Some yoga poses may feel fun and easy to access while others are more challenging. I often hear people say things like "I'm not flexible, so I don't do yoga" or "I can't touch my toes, so I don't do yoga." So often the images of yoga practitioners in the media are of very flexible people doing challenging poses upside down and sideways or twisting in ways that might seem impossible to the everyday practitioner. Fear not, yoga really is for everyone. If your kid has tight hamstrings, they can bend their knees as much as they'd like in order to reach a simpler version of a Forward Fold (page 42). There is no goal in yoga other than to be present with yourself and connect to what is true for you.

There are over 100 yoga activities to explore in this book, providing plenty of variety for you and your family. The poses are broken down into standing poses, seated poses, bends and twists, and balancing poses. Every pose and activity provides a new physical and mental adventure.

GAMES

Yoga games provide a fun entry point for the young budding yogi. They help kids practice yoga poses while building excitement and a sense of unity. These are a wonderful starting point for younger children especially, and fun for the whole family. Chapter 10 (page 169) offers easy-to-learn yoga games to keep your yoga time interesting.

SEQUENCES

A yoga sequence is a series of poses designed to guide the body through the practice. Sequences can take on various qualities depending on the teacher and mode of yoga being practiced: short or long, fast or slow, calming or energizing. When you and your child discover a yoga sequence that works for you, allow it to become your go-to yoga routine. You can also add to it or mix it up any time. Jason Crandell, one of my yoga teachers, often reminds his students that simple, repeatable postures have the most powerful and soothing effect on the body. Yoga works best when it's practiced frequently and honestly, in a way that nourishes you.

RELAXATION

In addition to movement, relaxation is an integral part of yoga. From Rest Pose (page 182) to guided meditations, a nourishing yoga practice includes moments of deep relaxation. Learning to unwind is crucial for adults and children. In yoga, we learn to anchor into the breath and consciously rest our bodies, which helps us release stress and find new reserves of energy. Yoga helps us recharge so we can peacefully approach the demands of daily life.

MEDITATION

Meditation is a powerful practice offering a variety of ways to tune into your thoughts and feelings. For kids, this is an influential and unique experience, as it is not something that is necessarily taught in schools or extracurricular activities. Meditation helps us notice our internal world without judgment. It's commonly practiced sitting still, but there are walking meditations and even meditations on eating! Meditation can be wonderfully calming and therapeutic some days, and it may feel excruciating on others.

It can be very difficult to slow down and sit still with so many distractions in today's world. However, encourage kids to keep trying even if they feel frustrated. One simple

STRUCTURING SESSIONS

Structuring a yoga class for the entire family may seem daunting at first, but with a little planning and persistence it can be a fun and rewarding experience. Using a combination of the yoga building blocks, practice what works best for you and your family. Most adult yoga classes take on the following form: meditation, breathing exercises, yoga sequences, and relaxation. Kid yoga classes are often structured differently for more engagement and interaction, depending on the age of your child.

Yoga sessions for kids tend to be shorter than the average one-hour classes offered at most yoga studios. In the beginning, getting in just three to five minutes of family yoga can be a big victory depending on your child's age and willingness to engage. These sessions are more playful and spontaneous than the average adult yoga class as well. They do not need to be quiet and reflective; you can talk, sing, guide, and delight in the poses and practice.

When first introducing yoga to young children, try to explain *why* you've decided to try this out as an activity together. Say something like "We're going to try yoga this morning to have fun and get ready for our day!" Or "We're going to practice something called yoga tonight to see if it helps us go to sleep easier." When you state the why with conviction, kids will gravitate toward the activity, even if they simply

watch you at first and do not practice along beside you. Modeling is incredibly powerful when it comes to mindfulness and yoga.

You might also build in various themes depending on what feels natural and meaningful to you and your child. If you know the teachers at your child's school are emphasizing gratitude, there are simple ways to weave this into a yoga session thematically. You could start the practice by appreciating that your body is healthy and able to engage in a yoga session. You could also encourage your child to imagine someone they appreciate in a meditation and later ask them why they appreciate that particular person.

Keep a flexible and open attitude when practicing yoga with kids. If you play just one yoga game before breakfast, congratulations! You've integrated yoga into your day. Longer sessions can include a variety of activities or simply one activity. If your child really enjoys active yoga poses but resists meditation or relaxation, start with sequences or choose a few poses to integrate every time you practice. The most important aspect of structuring a family yoga practice is to be present to your child's needs and preferences.

but effective way to help kids notice the power of meditation is to ask them how they feel on a scale of 1 to 10 before and after the meditation. This simple inquiry helps kids notice the effects of the meditation without too much probing or discussion. Meditators have long claimed that the practice helps them feel more calm, focused, and peaceful. A recent study led by a team of Harvard scientists at Massachusetts General Hospital revealed that in just eight weeks of regular meditation, gray matter density decreased in the amygdala region of the brain—an area responsible for stress and anxiety. "It is fascinating to see the brain's plasticity and that, by practicing meditation, we can play an active role in changing the brain and can increase our well-being and quality of life," says Britta Hölzel, first author and research fellow.

AGE CONSIDERATIONS

Practicing yoga with children can look very different depending upon their ages. Sometimes it can be a challenge to work with multiple age groups at once, but the trick is in variety and teamwork. Let yoga be a way for both older and younger kids to build their leadership and teamwork skills.

AGES 3 TO 4

These youngsters are developing a sense of imagination in leaps and bounds and need quick, playful activities. Use songs and games with this age group. Song can be interwoven into yoga poses in a few ways. If you and your child respond to music during yoga, play some favorites as background music to set the tone for your session. You can also sing songs as you practice yoga. You might sing a few rounds of "Row, Row, Row Your Boat" as you practice Boat pose (page 94) or wiggle your fingers and sing "Twinkle, Twinkle Little Star" as you hold Star pose (page 64). You can also get creative with your little one, making up songs with them as you move, stretch, breathe, and play.

You can also make up your own stories, use stories that are familiar, or use a few of the stories offered later in this book (see pages 176–179). Use everyday objects in your home to entice your toddler—an imaginary bubble can become a creative prop instantly when you "toss" it into the air and ask your child to take a big deep breath and observe it as it floats to the ground. Kids of this age respond well to adults pretending to be silly with imaginary objects. In daily life, assist your toddler in gaining mindfulness skills by helping her understand how she feels. When she is happy, ask her how it feels. When she is sad or angry, help her notice these emotions but remind her of the happy feelings she experienced in the past.

Toddlers enjoy the basic poses like Down Dog (page 52) (bark like a dog with them if they enjoy the noise!) and Bridge (page 60). They are also able to feel mastery with standing poses like Mountain (page 40) and Star (page 64). Partner poses like Airplane (page 160) or Double Boat (page 164) are easy and fun with this age group.

Limit yoga sessions with young toddlers to 15 minutes (which I'd call ambitious!), and consider it an accomplishment if you get in 5 minutes. Find ways to engage your young child by asking her to unroll the yoga mat or be in charge of the "Peaceful Spray" (see page 21).

AGES 5 TO 6

Five- and six-year-olds thrive on creativity and storytelling. Music still makes a big impression on these youngsters, so continue using songs. Call-and-response can be a fun and effective way of initiating yoga time. This can be as simple as saying the name of the pose as you transition into it. For instance, you say "Mountain" and your child repeats "Mountain" as they try the pose. You can do this in a straightforward way using a regular voice, or mix it up depending on the mood you are trying to create, with a whisper for a more calming effect or a silly voice to infuse more laughter and joy.

Many yoga poses are appealing to this age group. Their balance and coordination are improving, so poses previously inaccessible or challenging, such as Half Moon (page 142) or Side Plank (page 144), now become possible.

This age group can focus for longer periods of time and even begin to use yoga and mindfulness strategies on their own without guidance. Engage them with new poses and play, and witness them integrate the benefits of yoga. As young as they are, this age group begins to understand and appreciate the way yoga makes them feel, so providing a little reflection and sharing time at the end of a session is a great idea.

AGES 7 TO 10

This age group is particularly attracted to challenges and teamwork. Turning activities into fun team challenges can work extremely well. Body awareness increases around this age, so your kids will enjoy movement and games. Try games like Yogi Twister (page 173) with this group, and don't be shy to incorporate partner poses. As motor skills, body awareness, and communication are generally more refined, kids of this age tend to do well with the more challenging partner poses, such as Double Plank (page 166), Double Dog (page 152), or Double Gate (page 162).

As children in this age bracket develop self-control, they are able to practice yoga for longer periods of time. Help them feel ownership of the practice by allowing them to choose activities, set timers, or pick out the music. This age group loves to be involved in setting the stage and the direction of an activity.

AGES 11 TO 12

Children in this age group are typically adapting to middle school culture. An emphasis on friendships is more present and peer pressure takes on new meaning. There tend to be more social stresses during this time.

With the onset of puberty, body image and awareness is also heightened for some children in this age group. Yoga is a soothing way to create positive connections to the body. It also provides a method for understanding the power of one's own thoughts and feelings, fostering individuality.

Emotions can run high during this time. Breathing activities, relaxation, and meditations are soothing and productive ways to regulate strong emotions and restore feelings of confidence and balance. Keep having fun and infusing joy into yoga practice with children of this age. The heightened ability to discern preferences might mean you get more resistance for adult-led activities. Go with the flow and work in routines with a strong emphasis on choice.

YOGA AT HOME (OR AT THE PARK, OR IN THE CAR)

Yoga can be done in the home or on the go. Breathing activities require no space and can be done anywhere. In addition to practicing together at home, mix it up by going to a park or the beach, or doing some exercises while driving in the car. The activities in this book can be done in all types of locations, and some are especially fun on family vacations or weekend outings.

WHEN TO PRACTICE

Yoga is beneficial at any time of the day, but it's important to look at the rhythms of your family life and integrate yoga time when it makes the most sense for your family. Morning yoga routines can establish a healthy and optimistic outlook for the day while building a sense of connection to one another. Evening routines can soothe and calm the nervous system and encourage a good night's sleep.

In the morning, the routine might look something like this: Breakfast, brush your teeth, yoga poses, breathing, and meditation, off to school or daily activity.

In the evening: Dinner, bath time, yoga poses, breathing and meditation, relaxation, bedtime.

After school: Snack time followed by yoga games or time to just play around with sequences or poses. Consider creating a fun after-school weekly schedule with Monday set aside for games, Tuesday for partner poses and meditation, Wednesday for relaxation, Thursday for yoga sequences, and a Friday fun day with kids' choice.

WHERE TO PRACTICE

Yoga can be practiced in any environment. It's important to be present to your surroundings and choose aspects of yoga that work in a safe way within the chosen space. Make sure clutter is cleared and everyone has enough room to practice.

You can create a safe and nurturing environment to practice yoga at home by removing distractions from the room, like screens, devices, or favorite toys. Many kids respond well to aromatherapy, so if you have a diffuser and some essential oils like lavender and eucalyptus, you can make a ritual out of turning on the diffuser before your sessions. If you will be focusing more on relaxation or meditation, dim the lights, play soothing music, and have cozy blankets and pillows on hand.

Try all different types of places for your yoga sessions. I've practiced headstands and handstands on the beach with my toddlers, which is more challenging, but also playful and fun. Breathing exercises can be done virtually anywhere. You might do a Bubble Breath (page 36) at a red light if you notice your kids (or yourself!) becoming impatient with traffic, or even on an airplane. Adapt to your surroundings and feel confident in trying activities in new places.

EQUIPMENT

Equipment for yoga is minimal. Yoga mats are nice to have but not necessary. When we travel, I typically just throw down a towel or blanket to practice. There are light travel yoga mats, but I rarely have space to pack even that!

Yoga blocks can also be useful as props to assist in building flexibility and ease in certain poses (for example, resting hands on blocks in a Forward Fold, page 42, if your child can't reach the ground). If you are not quite ready to make the investment in yoga blocks, you can also stack a few sturdy books and use the book stack to assist you or your child in certain poses. A yoga strap can come in handy for stretching poses, but isn't essential.

For very young children around ages two to five, I also like to use tape to block the yoga mat into quadrants. This helps kids as you instruct them and assists them in building their spatial awareness as it relates to yoga activities.

It can also be nice to have what I call "Peaceful Spray" for your yoga practice. To make this, I add a few drops of essential oil to water in a misting bottle and spray it at the beginning of practice or during meditation to help calm the mind.

TIPS

In my years doing yoga with children of all ages, I've discovered some tips for creating the most fulfilling family practice.

Keep yoga time joyful and playful. The more you exude a love of yoga, the more your child will respond to the practice. Smile and laugh and bring humor to the activities. Celebrate effort and success and guide activities with optimism.

Start where you are. Keep your yoga practice simple and straightforward. Practice the activities you gravitate toward most naturally. If some days it seems you or your child need more nurturing, opt out of the poses and focus on relaxations and meditations. These count just as much as the more physical poses. Every day, try to be present to your needs and the needs of your child. Take it one breath at a time.

Make it routine. Building a yoga routine into the day helps you and your child anticipate yoga time like any other activity. Even toddlers enjoy knowing what comes next. Consider building in routines at specific times of day like morning, afternoon, or bedtime. Yoga can also be a routine before or after every game, competition, or recital. Allow yoga routines to make sense with the specific rhythms of your children and household. Provide opportunities for your child to influence and take responsibility for yoga time.

Use questions and adapt. As you guide yoga sessions, use questions. If you notice your child seems uncomfortable, ask him how he feels. Encourage him to connect and reflect, building self-awareness and a mind-body connection. Be flexible with activities and routines. If something isn't working, give yourself freedom to stop, move on, and try again another time. Bringing confidence and your own sense of flexibility to the practice encourages children to do the same.

Model kindness. Modeling kindness in yoga is one of the most powerful aspects of the practice. Yoga encourages us to slow down and be kind to ourselves and others. Say kind things to children while they practice, and be kind to yourself as you try new poses and activities. Children will make the connection between yoga and kindness and feel inspired to carry it into the world.

Think out loud. Narrate your experience as well as what you're witnessing with the rest of the group practicing yoga together. You can talk during yoga time! Connecting to the breath and silence is great but not always possible when practicing yoga with children. Model awareness with phrases like "Oh, wow. I just noticed my knee hurts in this Forward Fold. I think I might be pushing myself a bit. I'm going to bend my knees and back off to see what happens." Or "That meditation was really challenging for me. I kept thinking about how the car broke down last night and we need to get it fixed. Taking deep breaths helped me relax even though my mind kept thinking about the car. What was meditation like for you today?"

Notice and name feelings. It's important for kids to reflect and track how they feel before and after yoga. This works for adults as well. Generally speaking, we feel better after practicing yoga and mindfulness. However, sometimes this may not be the case. For example, we may be agitated or just moving through life so quickly that we aren't taking time to notice how we're feeling. Sometimes when we create the space for quiet, meditation, and even connecting to our breath, we may actually come into closer contact with feelings that may be deemed uncomfortable, like sadness or anger. It's okay! Understand that as you notice these feelings and make space for them to emerge, you are no longer repressing them and that's a very good thing. Let your children know that anything they feel during and after yoga is perfectly okay.

ALL ABOUT SAFETY

With a few necessary precautions, yoga is a safe and low-risk activity to engage in your home or on the go. It's important to stick to the following guidelines:

- **Don't push it.** Please be gentle with yourself and your child as you engage in yoga activities. No yoga pose is worth injury or pain. If you notice your child striving to get into a pose that is not accessible, please encourage her to back off and try a simpler version of the pose. Remind her that with practice, all will come. A good rule of thumb is that if you can't take a deep breath in a pose, you're probably pushing it too hard.

- **Mind the physical space.** Make sure the yoga space is clear of objects that might cause anyone harm. An easy gauge is to use Star pose (page 64), with arms and legs extended wide, to make sure that you won't bump into any furniture, other household items, or each other. This is important especially with yoga games, which may require more activity or space.

- **Press pause.** If you witness your child becoming unruly or moving his body in an unsafe way during a yoga session, stop whatever you're doing and take a pause. Sometimes kids may act silly or overextend themselves, especially when an activity is new. Remember that there is no harm in pausing and starting over or trying again the next day. This demonstrates to your child that safety is most important when we're practicing yoga and mindfulness.

GETTING KIDS INVOLVED

For most kids, yoga is a foreign concept. When you introduce yoga to your kids and they demonstrate reluctance or even defiance, you may be tempted to give up. In my experience leading yoga and mindfulness programs in K–12 schools, many of the students most deeply impacted by the practice are those who were initially most reluctant. Keep in mind that sitting still and connecting with feelings may be scary and new to some kids, and acting out is a natural (and sane!) reaction.

If you meet some resistance, reflect on simple changes you might make to the yoga routine to engage your child or to provide her with some ownership of the session. Ask her if she'd like to lead a pose or use the "Peaceful Spray" (see page 21) before you begin. Try shortening the yoga session, or giving her other activity options to choose from.

Remember that yoga is an activity you're offering to kids because you understand the incredible benefits. Just like eating healthier foods, they may not take to it immediately. Keep your offerings short and sweet to begin with, and once you notice more engagement, increase the time in small increments.

HIT THE MAT!

It's time to get started! With over 100 options, from breathing exercises and meditations to poses, sequences, and games, this book provides plenty to keep kids engaged and learning.

On any given day, yoga practice looks and feels different. One day your child might be thrilled to try some yoga poses and the next day she might say it's boring or she hates it. Kids can be so much more honest than adults. Push through any resistance by

SIBLING PRACTICE

Many children take to yoga practice naturally and will delight in teaching yoga to siblings, friends, and other family members. Although this book is meant to encourage yoga activities for kids and parents, kids can engage with the poses with their siblings or friends, too. They can use the illustrations and activities as a guide, or you can help them create a "pose chart" so they can point to a pose and show siblings and friends.

Partner poses and games can be a great way for kids to interact with one another, whether during a playdate with friends or just some downtime on a Sunday with siblings. Encourage your child to engage with other kids in a safe and kind way when introducing yoga, and be sure to keep a close eye on them.

acknowledging and accepting your child's feelings and providing other options for her. If she doesn't want to meditate, try a yoga game instead. The power of choice can make a big difference.

To help you get started, here are a few ideas for structuring a practice:

1. Yoga game, yoga poses, yoga sequence, relaxation
2. Breathing practice, meditation, relaxation
3. Yoga poses, yoga sequence, game, breathing practice
4. Relaxation, meditation, yoga sequence, breathing practice, relaxation
5. Yoga sequence, meditation, yoga sequence, meditation

No matter what happens, don't forget to feel proud of your efforts. You are teaching your child to build positive mind-body habits, which will serve her on and off the mat. Every little moment practicing yoga or mindfulness helps, so be sure to give yourself credit for sharing this amazing tool with your loved ones.

3

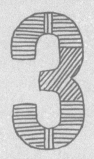

BREATHING EXERCISES

Many of us have been offered the advice "take a deep breath" when we feel stressed out and overwhelmed, but how many of us remember to do this of our own volition? We've probably offered this advice to our children when they're crying, anxious, or in the middle of a tantrum. In yoga, breathing activities are designed to calm the nervous system by working to activate the parasympathetic nervous system, one of the body's systems that keeps us feeling rested and calm. One of the most powerful aspects of yoga and mindfulness is the connection and awareness we create in relationship to our breath. We begin to notice when our breath is shallow or quick and we receive signals about our stress levels more easily. Taking a moment to slow down and breathe helps us experience life's challenges and joys.

PEACE BEGINS WITH ME

ALL AGES

 REJUVENATING

I learned this breathing practice from Ms. Jones and her second-grade students at Rooftop Elementary School in San Francisco. They use this breath daily to unify the classroom and transition from one activity to the next. It's easy to do at any time of day and fills the body and mind with a positive and grounding affirmation.

1. Slow down your breathing by taking nice, deep, slow breaths.

2. After a few rounds of deep breathing, press your pinky to your thumb.

3. Take a big inhale and on the exhale alternate consecutive fingers as you say the following words: "Peace (pinky), begins (ring) with (middle), me (forefinger to thumb)."

4. To slow it down, take another deep breath in and out through the nose after saying "me."

5. Practice a few rounds and focus on the rhythm of the words.

6. Try again silently, saying the words to yourself in your head.

BALLOON BREATH

ALL AGES

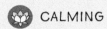 CALMING

This is a go-to breathing exercise that helps bring awareness to the breath in a simple and fun way. The metaphor of the balloon encourages kids to expand the breath on the inhale and let it go on the exhale. This may sound simple, but often when kids take a deep breath, they suck their tummies in on the inhale. A more calming effect happens when the belly expands on the inhale and relaxes on the exhale. You can practice Balloon Breath while sitting, lying down, or even standing.

1. Inhale gently through your nose, blowing your belly up like a balloon for a count of 1-2-3.

2. Exhale through your mouth, exhaling the air from the balloon, counting 3-2-1.

3. Imagine the color of your balloon and visualize it as you take a few more rounds of balloon breath.

4. Repeat three to five times, or as many times as you'd like.

TIP

- For an extra challenge, set a timer for three to five minutes and ask everyone to practice Balloon Breath on their own until the timer goes off.

WE GOT THIS

ALL AGES

 REJUVENATING

This is a partner exercise that deepens our connection with others. While practicing the breath, you feel the support of each other by holding each other up. This reminds us that we're in it together, and we've got each other's backs no matter what!

1. Sit down back-to-back on the floor with legs crossed and backs slightly touching.

2. Tune into your own body and breathing first. Notice how you feel as you slow your breath down.

3. Now shift your attention to your partner.

4. Notice the physical support of your partner.

5. Take an inhale, and on the exhale say silently "We got this."

6. Repeat three to five times or as many times as you'd like.

7. To infuse more energy into this breathing exercise, do a few rounds saying "We got this" together aloud.

TIP

- If you have an odd number of people, try one group of three in a triangle with their shoulders touching instead of backs.

FLOWER BREATH

ALL AGES

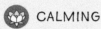 CALMING

This breathing exercise keeps little (and big!) hands moving while breathing and is great to use when it feels tough to sit still. As you practice Flower Breath with children, you can explain that every living thing is connected to the breath; even flowers need oxygen to breathe. It also encourages creative visualization, which is a useful technique in meditation.

1. Take a couple of slow, deep breaths in through the nose and out through the mouth.

2. Cup your hands so that all your fingers cup in toward the thumbs.

3. Inhale through the nose.

4. Exhale out through the mouth, opening the fingers and thumb, to allow the flower to "bloom."

5. Activate the imagination by envisioning a particular type of flower, the color of its petals, or even imagine its fragrance.

6. Close the hands to inhale, and on the exhale, open the hands again.

7. Do three to five rounds of Flower Breath.

8. When finished, ask everyone to describe their flowers.

COUNTING BREATH

ALL AGES

 SOOTHING

 CONCENTRATION

Similar to Balloon Breath (page 29), this practice is simple and soothing. Counting produces a calming and therapeutic effect when paired with deep breathing. The simplicity of counting gives the mind a predictable pattern and helps build focus and concentration. For variation, try counting in different languages.

1. Match your breathing with simple counting.

2. Take a deep inhale and then exhale, counting 1. Inhale again and exhale, 2. The numbers can be stated aloud, or instruct everyone to count silently.

3. Keep going for as many rounds as you'd like.

TIP

- Get creative! You don't have to just count up from 1. Try counting backward from 100. Or start with a specific number. For instance, if your child is turning seven soon, you might say "Let's start with seven. I love that number."

LION'S BREATH

ALL AGES

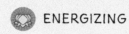 ENERGIZING

Fun for adults and kids alike, Lion's Breath is playful and refreshing. This is a great breath to practice if you feel emotional or angry, because it offers a sense of relief. Invite your children to release their anger or frustration with a Lion's Breath at any point during a yoga session or while out in the world.

1. Take a big breath into your belly and reach your arms over your head like a roaring lion.

2. Open your fingers wide, palms facing the front of your yoga mat.

3. As you exhale, push the air out of your belly and stick out your tongue, making a loud sound emulating a lion's roar. Simultaneously pull your arms down by your side, hugging the elbows in by the rib cage, hands up with fingers open wide.

4. Repeat as many times as you'd like.

"I AM" BREATH

ALL AGES

 SOOTHING

This breath is a wonderful way to integrate the power of affirmations into a physical exercise. You'll choose a quality to invite into your life—some examples include love, peace, calm, and strength. This quality will be your intention for the breathing exercise. To promote connection and support, share your intention with others in your practice and encourage them to do the same. Hearing the intentions of others gives us a glimpse into their internal world and fosters empathy.

1. Choose a quality to invite into your life—this is the intention for your practice.

2. As you inhale, say to yourself "I am."

3. As you breathe out, say the particular quality you want to cultivate.

4. For example, inhale "I am" and exhale "love."

5. Repeat a few times.

6. Notice how you feel, and draw on this breath any time you feel disconnected from your chosen quality.

BREATH OF JOY

ALL AGES

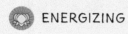 ENERGIZING

This breath is a fun and energizing way to get the day started. This breathing exercise is natural for kids (and adults) who may have a hard time sitting still and need a more active entry point into breathing exercises. It makes a great homework break or pre-game activity to help release the jitters.

1. Stand with your feet solidly on the ground. Make sure you have plenty of space around you for safety.

2. Start with your arms by your side.

3. Simultaneously swing your arms front and back by your sides while saying "Breathe in, breathe in."

4. On the third instruction to breathe in, reach your arms up high overhead.

5. Say "Breathe out."

6. As you exhale, say "Ahhhhhhhh" and fold over the legs, allowing your weight to tumble toward the ground in a Forward Fold (page 42).

7. After a few slow breaths, roll the spine back up to standing.

8. Repeat as many times as you'd like.

TIP

- Ask your child to share how he's feeling with one simple word before Breath of Joy. Afterward, ask him the same question. You can ask him why he thinks this is called Breath of Joy. Another way to integrate more connection is to ask him what brought him joy in his day. If you practice this pose in the morning, ask him to anticipate what will bring him joy.

BUBBLE BREATH

ALL AGES

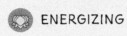 ENERGIZING

Bubble Breath appeals to your child's sense of imagination and is useful in situations that require kids to be quiet. It's a great way to find silence without shushing your child or saying "be quiet!" Plus, children really have fun with this one—a win-win!

1. Ask everyone in the session to get ready to "catch an imaginary bubble."

2. Pretend you are tossing a bubble their way with your hands.

3. Demonstrate how to puff out both cheeks in an exaggerated way in order to "catch" it.

4. Now "pop the bubble" and exhale out the mouth.

TIP

• Use variations with your language and body actions to promote imagination and make the exercise more playful. For example, you could say "Okay, are you ready for a gigantic bubble this time? Oh, it's so big I can barely hold it up with my hands!" Pretend the bubble is weighing you down to the ground and that you can barely find the strength to toss it.

BUMBLEBEE BREATH

ALL AGES

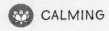 CALMING

This breathing exercise looks a little silly, but don't be afraid to embrace the silliness! This exercise is also calming and soothing to the nervous system. Despite the noise and initial giggles, the effects are quite grounding. This breath is wonderful when you're feeling overwhelmed or emotional. And it's no surprise that it's also a hit with kids.

1. Close your eyes if you'd like. (I always invite kids to close their eyes rather than making it a command.)

2. Inhale through your nose as you plug each ear with your fingers.

3. As you exhale, make a humming sound that buzzes like a bumblebee.

4. Keep buzzing for about a minute, holding the exhale for as long as possible and inhaling and exhaling as necessary.

5. Repeat as many times as you'd like.

TIP

- Use Bumblebee Breath as an opportunity to discuss symbiotic relationships in nature. Depending on your child's age, you can simplify or expand the conversation. Even three-year-olds are fascinated by nature's simple lessons.

CHAPTER

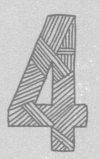

4

BASIC POSES

Yoga is built from a foundation of basic poses. Build your yoga practice as you first learn to move your body into these poses. You and your kids will find these poses crop up again and again in your yoga sequences, so it's helpful to get comfortable with them early on. Practicing just a few of these poses a day will help build a lasting yoga habit in your household.

MOUNTAIN

ALL AGES

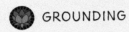 GROUNDING

At first glance, Mountain pose may simply look like standing, but really it is so much more! Help kids feel as strong as a mountain by emphasizing strong legs, a long spine, relaxed shoulders, and hands active by their sides. Mountain pose is the starting point for many yoga sequences and is a great pose to come back to if little ones get distracted during practice.

1. Start by standing with your feet hip-width apart.

2. Take a slight bend in your knees.

3. Gradually straighten the legs, pointing your tailbone down toward the ground.

4. Take a deep inhale and imagine you are getting longer through your spine.

5. Exhale and relax your shoulders by gently drawing the shoulder blades down the back.

6. Relax your hands by your sides, palms facing forward with fingers spread wide.

7. Breathe deeply a few times, standing tall and confident.

TIPS

- Try this pose with your eyes closed and encourage kids to notice how strong and tall they feel.
- To make it more fun, name everyone in the room as a mountain. For instance, you could say "Wow, you look like Mt. Olivia now!"
- This pose can be a great tool out in the world as well. Ask children to "be a mountain" when you need them to be still, safe, and quiet while in public places or hectic situations.

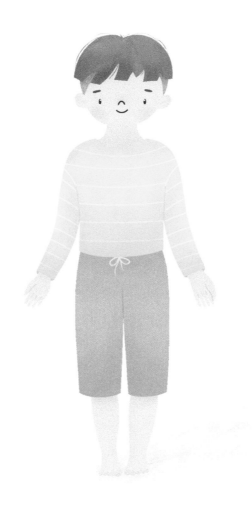

FORWARD FOLD

ALL AGES

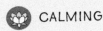 CALMING

Forward Fold increases blood flow to the heart and head. It also improves lower-body flexibility and provides a great release in the lower back. This is a great pose to incorporate early on in your practice to get the blood flowing. Encourage kids to notice how Forward Fold feels at the beginning of practice and later on when the muscles have warmed up some—chances are, they'll find themselves bending even deeper toward the ground.

1. Start in Mountain pose (page 40).

2. Take a slight bend in your knees.

3. Press your feet down into the ground and raise your arms over your head.

4. Take a deep inhale and, as you exhale, slowly dive down toward the floor, keeping your spine long as you lower down.

5. While in Forward Fold, take a few deep breaths and let your head hang down.

6. To release the pose, place your hands on your hips and slowly lift up, keeping your spine long and using your core to lift you up to standing.

TIPS

- If your hands don't touch the floor, bring the floor to you! Use yoga blocks or stacks of books under your hands for additional support.
- While folded, try grabbing opposite elbows and swaying gently from side to side. This helps the head and neck release while stretching the lower back.

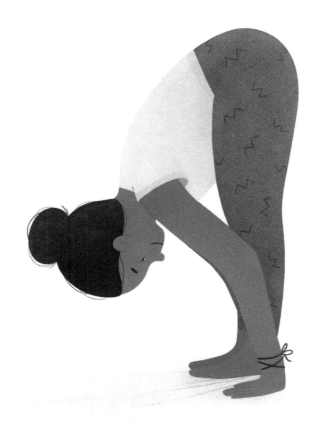

TABLE TOP

ALL AGES

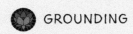 GROUNDING

Table Top pose is a foundational resting pose we often use between poses. Be sure to keep your core engaged and neck long while in this pose. Encourage kids to make their back "as flat as a table" while in this position—you could even try balancing something light on their backs to make it more fun.

1. Set your knees and hands down on the yoga mat.

2. Line up your wrists directly beneath your shoulders and your knees under your hips.

3. Press your hands down firmly into the ground.

4. Elongate your spine.

5. To keep the neck long, focus your gaze on a spot just in front of the hands in the center of the yoga mat.

6. Take a few deep breaths, feeling your body strong and active in the pose.

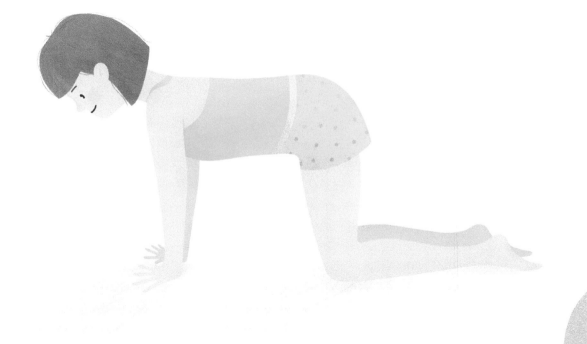

CHILD'S POSE

ALL AGES

 CALMING

 GROUNDING

Child's Pose is an important resting pose in yoga. Encourage self-care in yourself and your little one by taking a break in Child's Pose whenever you need to rest and regroup. You can take the pose at any time during a yoga session or during a stressful moment in your day. Resting the forehead on the ground with the head lower than the heart has a restorative and calming effect. You can remind kids that they loved this pose when they were babies, before they even knew what yoga was!

1. Start in Table Top (page 44).
2. Take your knees wide and bring your big toes together to touch, if possible.
3. Press down with your hands and push your body back and down between your thighs.
4. Keep your arms reaching forward, resting on the yoga mat.
5. Let your forehead rest on the mat, staying long through the spine.
6. Take slow, deep breaths as you feel the weight of the body completely taken by gravity. Relax the neck and shoulders even as the hands press into the ground.
7. To release, slowly lift the upper body into a seated position on your heels, or another comfortable seated position that works for you.

TIP

- Add in gentle movement by trying some Child's Pose to Table Top (page 44) stretches. From Child's Pose, inhale and lift up and forward into Table Top. On the exhale, send the body back into Child's Pose. Repeat and experience a rocking, therapeutic sensation as you match the breath with your movements.

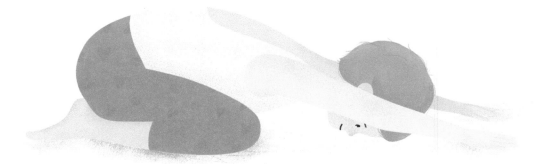

CAT

ALL AGES

 CALMING

 REJUVENATING

In Cat, we round the spine high and tall. This stretches the back, shoulders, and neck. Be sure to let your head hang heavy to take pressure off the neck. When you exhale into Cat, squeeze the belly in as far as it will go and round the spine at the same time. You can even say "squeeeezzze" to encourage everyone to exhale and squeeze the belly in.

1. Start in Table Top (page 44).

2. Take a deep inhale and on the exhale, arch your spine (like a cat) toward the ceiling as you tuck your chin in toward your chest.

3. Exhale all the air out and hold the pose for a moment before you make your way back into Table Top. Take a few deep breaths.

TIP

- With young children, try working in a "meow" or "hiss" with this pose.

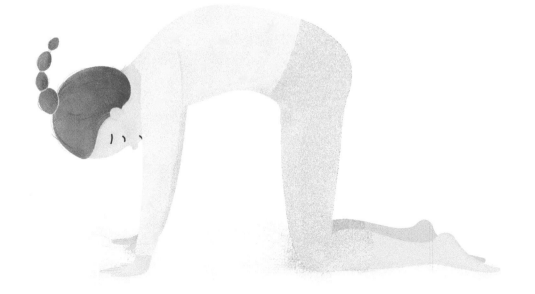

COW

ALL AGES

 CALMING

 REJUVENATING

Cow pose is a slight adjustment to Table Top (page 44), and the counterbalance to Cat (page 48). In Cow, we stretch the belly down toward the earth and open the heart up to the sky. Encourage kids to look "up, up, up!" to get the best stretch through the neck and shoulders.

1. Start in Table Top (page 44).
2. Take a deep inhale and exhale.
3. On your next inhale, drop your chest and belly down toward the floor as you lift your chin and gaze up to the sky.
4. Draw your shoulder blades down the back. Hold the inhale as long as you can.
5. Exhale to release the pose and make your way back into Table Top.

TIP

- Combining Cat and Cow together is known as "Cat-Cow" and is a satisfying mini-sequence. Inhale for Cat and exhale for Cow, repeating as many times as you'd like. Tell kids to "meow" and "moo" as they keep breathing and stretching.

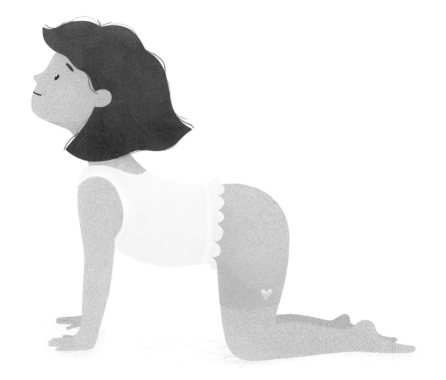

DOWN DOG

ALL AGES

 REJUVENATING

Down Dog is a simple inversion and a basic building block for yoga sequences. Young kids love this one because they can pretend to be a dog while trying out the pose. While Down Dog is simple, you can always continue to refine the position by pressing down with your fingers, sending your hips up higher, rotating your elbows in, and pressing your heels toward the mat. Nearly the whole body is engaged during this pose.

1. Start in Table Top (page 44).
2. Press your hands into the ground, fingers spread wide.
3. Lift your knees off the ground and send your hips high into the air toward the ceiling, forming an upside-down "V" shape with the entire body.
4. Press your hands and feet firmly into the ground as the spine elongates and the neck and head relax.
5. Soften your gaze between your feet.
6. Take a few deep breaths. Return to this pose whenever you need to.

TIPS

- For children ages two to nine, ask them to "wag their doggie tail" and "bark like a dog" while in the pose to make it more playful and engaging.
- Invite your child to wiggle on her belly underneath your Down Dog in order to go "through the tunnel."

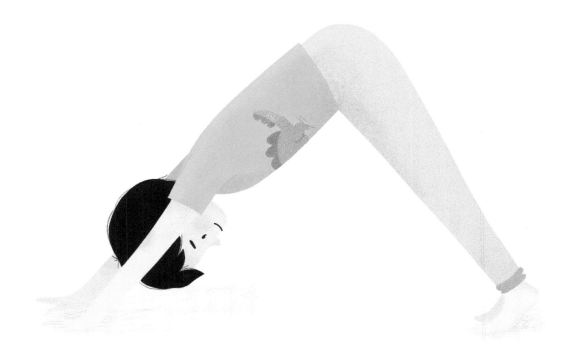

PLANK

ALL AGES

 STRENGTHENING

Plank is also commonly called "top of a push-up" because it is the strong, straight position you assume before lowering into a push-up. Plank pose is challenging, firing up the core, shoulders, and upper arms. Many kids enjoy the challenge of holding Plank. Try counting aloud together as you hold this position.

1. Start in Down Dog (page 52).

2. Press your hands and feet into the ground and engage the core muscles.

3. Glide forward until your shoulders are directly over your hands.

4. Press firmly into the ground with your hands, fingers spread wide.

5. Keep the upper back lifted between the shoulders.

6. Press back with the heels, lifting up with your thighs.

7. Take a deep inhale and exhale. Hold for as many breaths as you'd like.

8. To release, bring the knees down to the floor into Table Top (page 44).

TIP

- To bring some movement into the pose, try moving back into Down Dog on the inhale and forward and down into Plank on your exhale. Repeat as many times as you'd like.

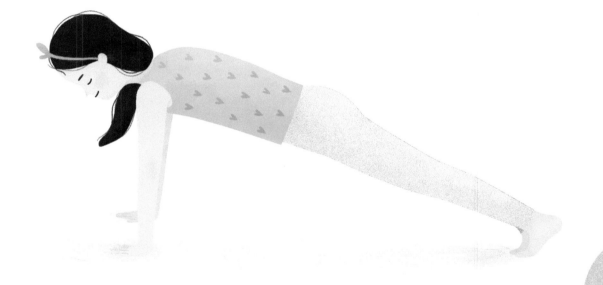

YOGA PUSH-UP

5 AND UP

 STRENGTHENING

A yoga push-up engages the core and upper arms and is all about alignment. This is a more challenging pose, so listen to your body and take your time with it. At first, allow the knees to stay on the floor while lowering the upper body down. This helps you build strength. Over time, your body will grow stronger and you will be able to lower with your knees off the floor. Remind kids to do what feels best for their body and have patience while practicing this pose.

1. Start in Plank (page 54).

2. Press your hands and toes firmly into the ground and engage your core muscles.

3. Inhale and glide forward slowly until your shoulders are slightly in front of your wrists and you are on your tippy toes.

4. Exhale and bend your elbows, keeping them tucked in by your ribs, and lower your body down a few inches.

5. To release, slowly lower your body to the floor and rest your head to one side, taking a deep breath in and out.

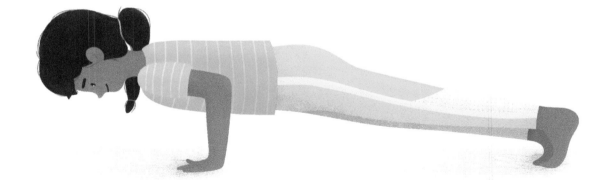

COBRA

ALL AGES

 HEART OPENING

Cobra is a gentle backbend that's integral to many yoga sequences but feels good practiced on its own as well. Kids love it because they get to pretend to be a snake while trying out this pose. Cobra stretches out the lower back and opens the heart and is foundational to other more strenuous backbends.

1. Start by lying facedown on the yoga mat with your upper body, belly, and legs pressing into the ground.

2. Place your hands on the mat directly underneath your shoulders, fingers spread wide.

3. Press the tops of your thighs and shins into the floor.

4. Breathing in, engage your core and lift your chest off the mat while keeping elbows bent and gently pressing your shoulder blades down your back.

5. Relax the neck and the face, and keep your gaze straight ahead.

6. To release, slowly lower the upper body down to the mat.

7. Turn your head to one side and take a few deep breaths, feeling the effects of the pose.

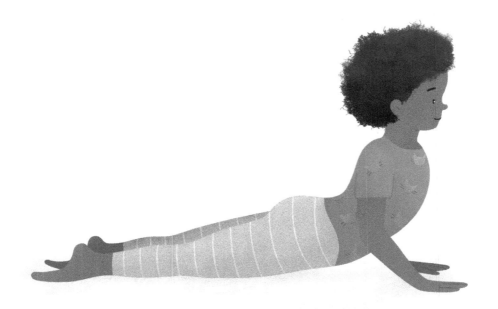

BRIDGE

ALL AGES

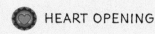 HEART OPENING

Bridge is a gentle backbend accessible for most children and adults. Tell kids to envision boats or trains running under their bridge so they press their hips up even higher. This pose stretches the back and neck and is foundational to other yoga backbends.

TIPS

- Bring movement into this pose by lifting the hips on the inhale and lowering the hips on the exhale. Repeat a few times.
- Play around with balance in Bridge pose. You can instruct your child to lift one foot off the ground just a few inches and hold it up in Bridge pose. Make sure to switch sides.

1. Start by lying on your back on the mat.

2. Bend your knees and draw your feet in toward your bottom with your feet directly under your knees.

3. Keep your hands by the sides of your thighs, palms facing down.

4. Inhale and relax your neck.

5. On the exhale, press your arms, hands, and feet firmly into the ground, engage the core and thighs, and raise the hips up until your thighs are parallel to the ground.

6. Lift the chin ever so slightly and choose a spot to look at to build focus.

7. Take a few deep breaths.

8. To release the pose, gently lower the hips to the ground and tuck the chin into the chest.

9. Place your hands on your belly with your knees still bent, and take a few deep breaths to feel the effects of the pose.

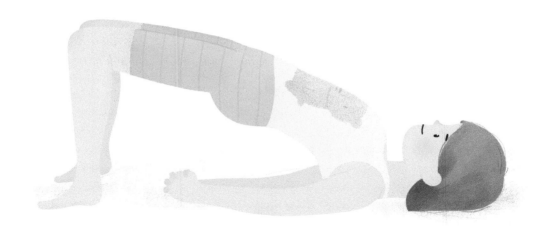

CHAPTER

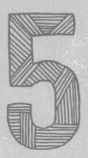

STANDING
POSES

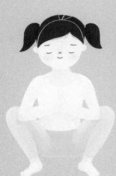
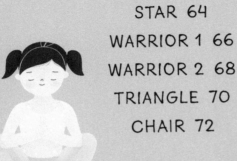

Standing poses are generally soothing to the nervous system and build strength in the legs. Kids especially enjoy the accessibility of standing poses. In all standing poses, an element of balance is required, helping kids and adults alike increase body awareness and stability. When engaging in standing poses, you can add in fun snaps and claps to build in rhythm and additional movement. Try Warrior 2 (page 68) with three snaps and claps, or sing "Twinkle, Twinkle" while holding Star pose (page 64).

STAR

ALL AGES

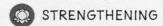 STRENGTHENING

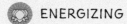 ENERGIZING

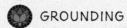 GROUNDING

Star is a fun and easy pose and a great way to kick off a yoga session with young children. It provides children with a sense of confidence and mastery and is foundational for accessing more complex poses like the Warrior poses (pages 66–69). Star pose comes alive when you shine your star outward by wiggling all of your fingers.

1. Step or hop your feet about three feet apart, depending on your height as well as your child's.

2. Keep both legs straight with toes facing forward.

3. Press your feet firmly into the ground.

4. Take a deep inhale and reach both arms out to the sides, stretching through your fingertips.

5. Exhale and relax your shoulders by gently drawing the shoulder blades down the back.

6. Breathe deeply a few times, standing strong and confident like a star.

TIP

- Star-Mountain is a wonderful pairing of poses and can evolve into a fun game. Simply guide your child into Star, and then ask her to jump into Mountain (page 40). Repeat. Then mix it up, trying different combinations like "Star. Star. Star. Mountain!" Have fun with it if she jumps into Mountain too soon. This simple activity also builds listening skills and focus.

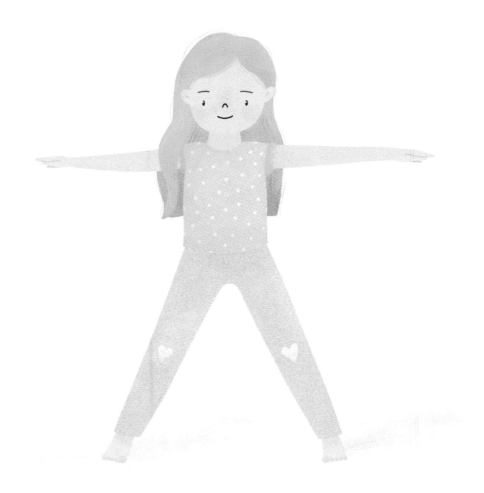

WARRIOR 1

5 AND UP

 STRENGTHENING

 GROUNDING

Warrior 1 is an integral standing pose for many yoga sequences. It calls on our inner strength and reminds us of our ability to overcome challenges. While in this pose, you'll root into the ground with your feet and simultaneously stretch your upper body toward the sky. Encourage kids to focus on these opposing sensations while holding the pose.

1. Begin in Mountain (page 40).

2. Step one foot back and bend the front knee to a 90-degree angle. Be sure that the bent knee does not go past the ankle. Turn the back foot out at a 45-degree angle.

3. If you find yourself losing balance, try doing the pose against a wall, pressing your back heel into the wall for added stability.

4. Angle the hips slightly forward to square them with the front of the room.

5. Press both feet firmly into the ground.

6. Take a deep inhale and lift both arms above your head.

7. Exhale and relax your shoulders and gently draw the shoulder blades down the back.

8. Breathe deeply, standing strong and confident.

9. To release, bring the back foot to meet the front foot, standing in Mountain.

10. Repeat on the other side.

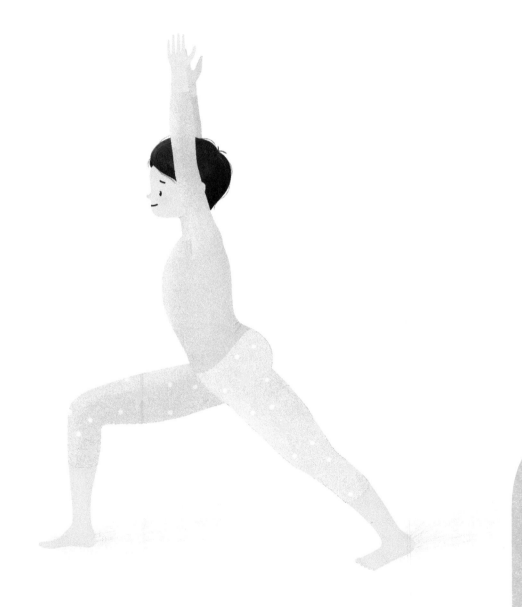

WARRIOR 2

5 AND UP

 STRENGTHENING

 GROUNDING

Warrior 2 builds strength in the legs and opens the heart. This pose is a great reminder that in order to be strong, we must also be kind, soft, and open to life's experiences. To keep little ones engaged in this pose, try adding snaps or claps while holding the pose.

TIP

- Play around with movement.
- On the inhale, extend the arms out and on the exhale draw the hands together at the sternum, clapping if your little one enjoys a bit more noise and excitement. Repeat a few times.
- Try more movement in the legs, too. On the inhale, straighten the front leg and on the exhale re-bend the knee, sinking back down into the pose.

1. Begin in Mountain (page 40).
2. Step one foot back and bend the front knee to a 90-degree angle. Make sure that the bent knee does not go past the ankle.
3. Turn the back foot out at a 45-degree angle, this time keeping your hips pointed to the side of the room.
4. If you find yourself losing balance, try doing the pose against a wall, pressing your back heel into the wall for added stability.
5. Press your feet firmly into the ground.
6. Take a deep inhale and reach both arms out to either side, stretching from the tips of your fingers.
7. Exhale and relax your shoulders by gently drawing your shoulder blades down the back.
8. Keep the front and back arms in a straight line, and gaze over your front middle finger.
9. Breathe deeply a few times, standing strong and confident.
10. To release, bring the back foot to meet the front foot, standing in Mountain.
11. Repeat on the other side.

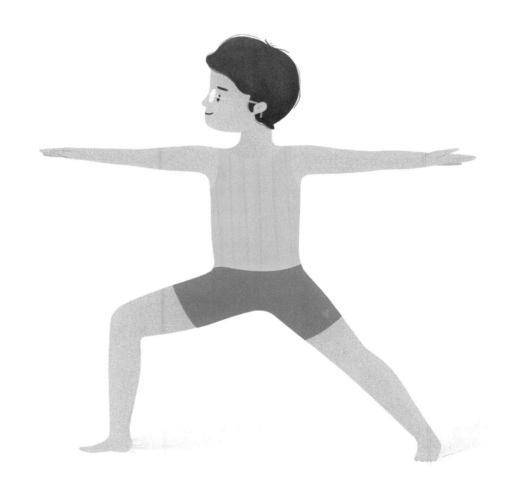

TRIANGLE

ALL AGES

 CALMING

 STRENGTHENING

Triangle pose is a great standing stretch that can be linked to teaching about shapes. The pose builds strength in the legs and flexibility in the hips and back. There's a lot going on in this pose, so it's helpful for concentration as well. Once you're in Triangle, try to keep your body flat as if you're between two panes of glass. This visualization will help you and your kids keep everything aligned.

TIPS

- Ask your child to show you how many triangles are actually in your triangle pose. (Hint: it's more than one!)
- Make a few simple arm movements while in Triangle. Circle the top arm around and down as you inhale and exhale, drawing large circles with the hand. Try a snap at the top of each circle.

1. Step or hop your feet about three feet apart, depending on your height as well as your child's.

2. Turn one foot out at a 90-degree angle, and turn your other foot in at a 45-degree angle.

3. Reach both arms out to either side.

4. Take a deep inhale and draw the front hip slightly back. Exhale as you reach the upper body as far as you can toward the front of the room. The back hip can move slightly forward to further extend the upper body.

5. Rest the front hand on your shin, ankle, a block, a stack of books, or the floor outside your front foot.

6. Reach the top arm straight up, palm facing forward.

7. Look toward the side of the room, or up toward the top hand if you feel balanced. If this bothers your neck at all, look down toward the front foot.

8. Take a few deep breaths.

9. To release, press both feet firmly into the ground and engage the core muscles as you lift your torso up to standing.

10. Repeat on the other side.

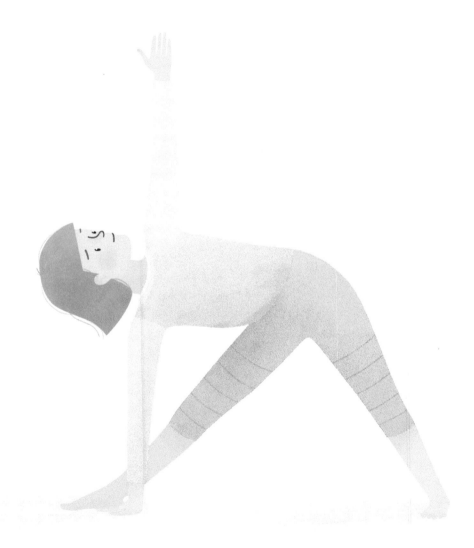

CHAIR

ALL AGES

 GROUNDING

 STRENGTHENING

Chair is a challenging pose. It builds strength in the legs and requires a lot of focus. At first it might be hard to hold this pose, but over time you will be able to sink deeper into your chair and hold it for longer. Encourage kids to use their imagination—maybe they are taking a seat in a race car or skiing down a mountain. The longer the ride, the longer they'll want to hold the pose.

1. Start in Mountain (page 40).

2. Bend both knees and engage the core muscles.

3. Reach the arms overhead.

4. Take a deep breath and imagine you are actually sitting down into a chair, sinking your hips down toward the floor as the upper body lifts. Direct your gaze to the floor slightly in front of you.

5. Relax your shoulders by gently drawing the shoulder blades down the back.

6. Breathe deeply a few times.

7. To release the pose, straighten your legs.

TIP

- Pretend you are skiing! Begin with the arms extended overhead as you inhale and then exhale— whoosh—as you send the arms back as if you're skiing. Make up a fun story about what you're seeing on the mountain along the way. Repeat a few times, straightening the legs if you or your child need a break.

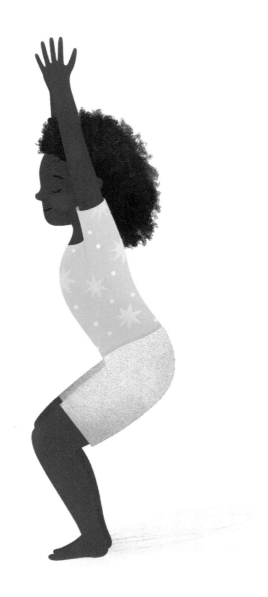

CANDLE

ALL AGES

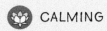 CALMING

Candle pose is a simple foundational pose for your yoga practice. It provides a steady way to integrate breath and movement into a yoga sequence. This is a great pose to use when your child needs to reset if he is very energetic or being silly with his body. This pose is especially soothing when integrated with movement and breath (see tip).

1. Place your knees hip-width apart on the yoga mat.

2. Inhale and press the palms together at your heart, lightly touching the thumbs to the sternum.

3. On the exhale, press the palms together, reach the arms overhead. If this causes any pain in the shoulders or neck, simply reach the arms straight up without pressing the palms together.

4. Take a deep breath and imagine you are a lit candle.

5. Relax your shoulders by gently drawing the shoulder blades down the back.

6. To release, gently drop the arms and sit back on your heels.

TIP

• Candle is a fun and easy way to get your child moving in the morning. As you inhale, say "light your candle" as she reaches her hands over her head. Next, say "blow out the candle" while instructing her to sit back on her heels, bring her hands back down in front of her, and exhale like she's blowing out a birthday candle. Move through this a few times to start off your day.

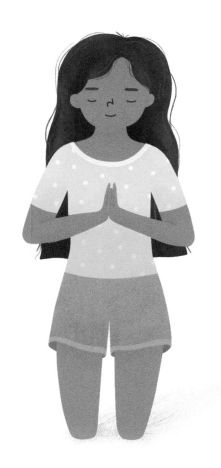

LOW LUNGE

ALL AGES

 GROUNDING

 CALMING

Low Lunge provides a deep stretch to the thigh muscles and hip flexors. It also provides some stability, as the knee stays planted on the ground in this pose. For extra protection and comfort, place a folded blanket underneath the knee. Low Lunge is a great precursor for the more challenging High Lunge (page 80).

1. Start in Candle (page 74).

2. Step one foot straight forward toward the front of the mat and bend the front knee to a 90-degree angle.

3. Inhale and lengthen the spine, taking both hands to the front thigh. Exhale here.

4. Inhale again and reach the arms up over your head, pressing firmly into the back foot.

5. Relax your shoulders by gently drawing the shoulder blades down the back.

6. Exhale and breathe deeply a few times, feeling length through the torso and arms and stability in the lower body.

7. To release the pose, return to Candle.

8. Repeat on the other side.

TIP

- To add some motion and heat here, bring both hands on either side of the front thigh and come onto the fingertips for extra length. Tuck the back toes so the toes press into the mat. On the inhale, gently lift the back knee up into a High Lunge (page 80). Set it back down to the mat on the exhale. Repeat.

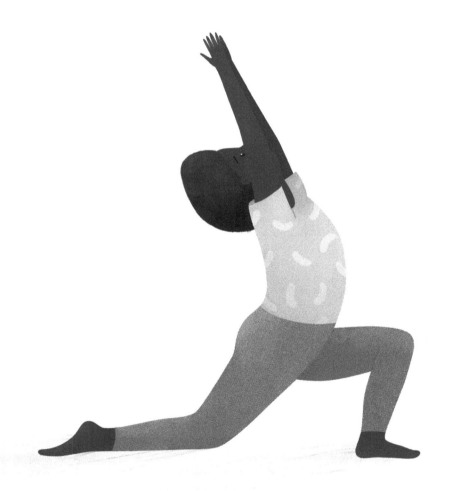

SIDE ANGLE

ALL AGES

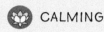 CALMING

Side Angle is a dynamic standing pose that strengthens the legs and stretches the side body. We focus on rooting down the lower body while lifting and stretching the upper body. Challenge everyone to make one long straight line with the side body while holding this pose.

1. Step or hop your feet about three feet apart, depending on your height as well as your child's.

2. Keep both legs straight. Turn your front foot out to a 90-degree angle and turn your back foot in slightly. Reach both arms out to the side.

3. Bend the front knee to a 90-degree angle.

4. Keep the hips pointing toward the side of the room. The back hip can move slightly forward in order to extend the upper body.

5. Rest the front arm lightly on your front thigh.

6. Pressing both feet firmly into the ground, reach the top arm straight up toward the ceiling, then extend it toward the front of the room over your ear.

7. Look toward the side of the room, or up toward the top hand if you feel balanced. If this bothers your neck at all, look down toward the front foot.

8. Take a few deep breaths.

9. To release, press the feet firmly into the ground and engage the core muscles to lift the torso to standing while straightening your front leg.

10. Repeat on the other side.

TIP

- Add more movement here by rotating between Side Angle and Warrior 2 (page 68). As you inhale, press into the feet and reach up and back into Warrior 2. As you exhale, extend back down into Side Angle. Repeat a few times.

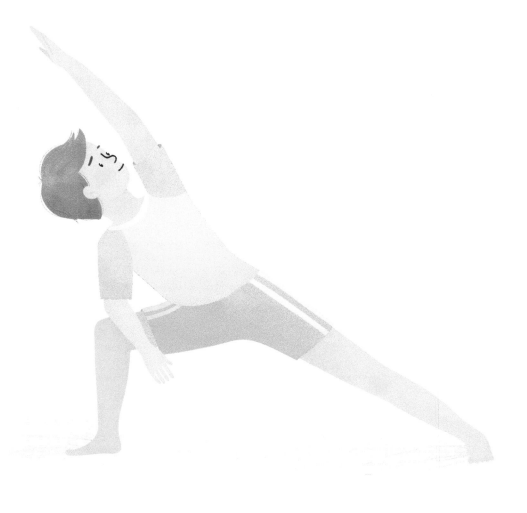

HIGH LUNGE

5 AND UP

 GROUNDING

 STRENGTHENING

High Lunge is a great way to stretch your quads and relieve tension in the hips. It also requires focus and balance. Squeeze your inner thighs together and reach your torso up to help bring more stability to the position. If you're feeling wobbly, you can always lower the back knee.

1. Start in Forward Fold (page 42).

2. Bend your knees. Pressing your fingertips into the ground, step the left foot back to the back of the yoga mat, keeping your left heel off the ground.

3. Lean your torso over the right thigh. If you feel balanced, try raising your torso to upright and lifting your arms straight up by your ears.

4. Press both feet into the ground, especially the ball of the left foot.

5. Relax your shoulders and gaze forward.

6. To release, place the left foot next to the right. Repeat on the second side.

TIP

• Create soothing movement by pressing the back knee to the ground on an inhale, and on the exhale, lifting back into High Lunge.

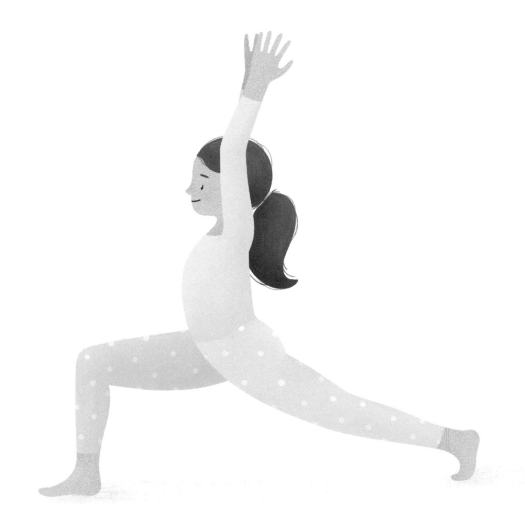

FROG

ALL AGES

 GROUNDING

 CALMING

Frog pose is an accessible hip opener that also stretches the ankles and back. Since this pose is a squat, it is a great counterbalance for adults and children who sit for long periods at a time during work or school. Make Frog more playful with "ribbits" and frog leaps and jumps. This is an all-around playful way to get started with a yoga practice.

TIPS

- From a squatting Frog position, you can ribbit your way into frog hops! Just make sure there is nothing in the way that could cause harm or injury.
- For an extra challenge, you can try leaping back into Yoga Push-Up (page 56) from Frog pose.

1. Step your feet apart wide enough so that you can squat your bottom down toward the ground, about the width of the mat. Turn your toes out slightly.

2. Inhale deeply. As you exhale, lower your bottom down as far as you can toward the ground. If you need additional support, try this against the wall. If your heels lift up, you can roll up a couple of towels and place them underneath your heels.

3. Press your palms together at your sternum and take a few deep breaths, opening the heart.

4. Take a deep breath and imagine that you are getting longer through your spine.

5. Relax your shoulders by gently drawing the shoulder blades down the back.

6. Breathe deeply a few times, feeling the support of the ground beneath you.

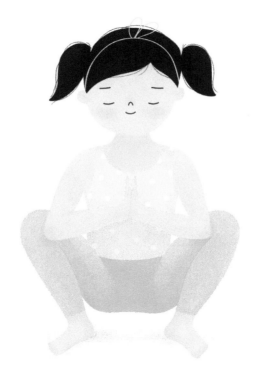

CHAPTER

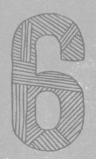

SEATED POSES

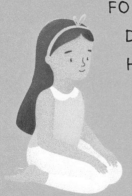

Seated yoga poses are grounding and calming and often improve flexibility through stretching. These poses are a great way to unwind with your child at the end of the day. Removing balance and strength from the equation, seated poses are a nice change of pace for the entire family. Seated poses also make it easier to focus on a steady rhythm with the breath. Build seated poses into your nighttime rituals or when you need a break from more active yoga poses.

BUTTERFLY

ALL AGES

 GROUNDING

 CALMING

Butterfly is a simple and fun seated pose. It's also a popular stretch in P.E. classes and other physical activities, so your kids are probably already familiar with the position. Focus on elongating the spine and relaxing the shoulders as you hold this pose. Over time, you'll notice increased flexibility. This seated pose is soothing and calming when done in a still way. Create more movement by "flapping your butterfly wings" or moving the legs gently up and down.

1. Start seated on the ground with your legs straight out in front of you.

2. Bend your knees outward and draw the soles of your feet together.

3. Bring your heels in toward the pelvis as far as feels comfortable for you. Let gravity pull your knees down toward the floor, and avoid actively pressing the knees down.

4. Take a deep breath and imagine growing longer through your spine.

5. Relax your shoulders by gently drawing the shoulder blades down the back.

6. Breathe deeply a few times, feeling the ground supporting you and a stretch through the spine and inner thighs.

TIPS

- With younger children, ages three to six, ask "What color is your butterfly?" while holding this pose.
- You can also have them flap their butterfly wings and then challenge them to keep their butterfly very still.

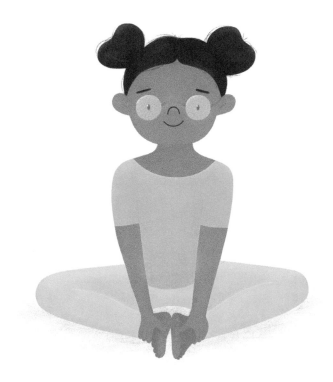

SEATED FORWARD BEND

ALL AGES

 GROUNDING

 CALMING

Seated Forward Bend is a wonderful pose to help you unwind and provide a moment of quiet stretching. It works well toward the end of a yoga session when muscles are warm and limber. Pay close attention to your breathing during this pose. If breathing stops or gets shallow, you're probably pushing it a little too hard. Remind kids that they can bend their knees as much as they need to as they fold over in the pose. The point is to get a nice long stretch in the legs and lower back.

1. Start seated on the ground with your legs straight out in front of you. It may be helpful to sit up on a folded blanket, so your hips are higher than your knees.

2. Gently press your fingertips down on either side of your hips as you press the legs into the mat. Take a deep inhale and elongate through the spine.

3. On the exhale, crawl your fingertips forward toward your feet, leaning forward as you go. Keep the spine straight and take slow, even breaths.

4. Lean forward as far as feels comfortable for you, making sure the spine stays long. Bend the knees slightly if it feels more comfortable. Do not force the body into going farther.

5. Relax your shoulders by gently drawing the shoulder blades down the back.

6. Take a few deep breaths in the fold.

7. To release, slowly lift up, keeping your spine straight.

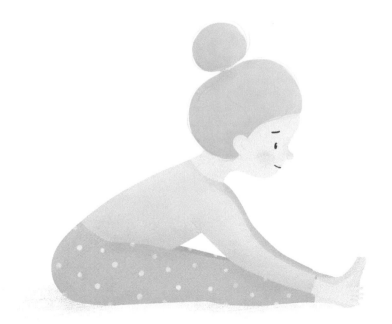

DRAGONFLY

ALL AGES

 GROUNDING

 CALMING

Dragonfly is also commonly called "head to knee" pose. This pose stretches the lower back and thighs and creates a calming opportunity to release the neck and shoulders in the fold. You can ask your child what color he wants his dragonfly to be and help him create a story about the dragonfly's whereabouts and adventures as you hold the pose steady.

1. Start seated on the ground with your legs straight out in front of you. It may be helpful to sit up on a folded blanket so your hips are higher than your knees.

2. Gently press your fingertips down on either side of your hips as you press the legs into the mat.

3. Draw one leg in, deeply bending the knee and pressing the sole of the foot against the opposite inner thigh.

4. Press into the fingertips and elongate the spine.

5. Slowly lean forward over the straight leg, keeping the spine long, and bending only to the point where you feel comfortable. You can slightly bend the extended knee if it feels more comfortable. Do not force the body into going farther.

6. Relax your shoulders by gently drawing the shoulder blades down the back.

7. Take a few deep breaths, growing long on the inhale, and melting into the fold on the exhale.

8. To release, inhale and rise back to a seated position, extending both legs out in front of you.

9. Repeat on the other side.

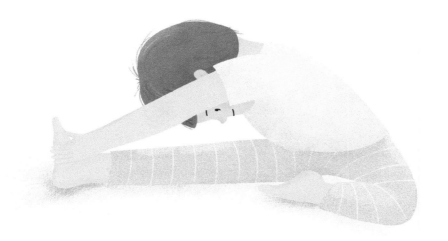

HAPPY BABY

ALL AGES

 GROUNDING

 CALMING

This sweet, playful pose releases the lower back and stretches the inner thighs. It's a bit of a silly pose, so be sure to embrace the silliness with your kids! You can have them make baby noises while rocking back and forth in the pose. Or, you might want to mention a special memory from when your child was a baby. This is a great pose for the end of a yoga session.

1. Start by lying on your back with your knees hugged in toward your chest.

2. Keeping the knees bent, grab the outer edge of your foot with the corresponding hand: right hand grabs outer edge of the right foot and left hand grabs outer edge of the left foot.

3. Allow your spine and lower back to release toward the ground, taking slow deep breaths.

4. If it feels comfortable and relaxing, rock from side to side in Happy Baby. Continue to breathe as you rock.

5. To release the pose, hug your knees back into your chest and make your way into a seated position.

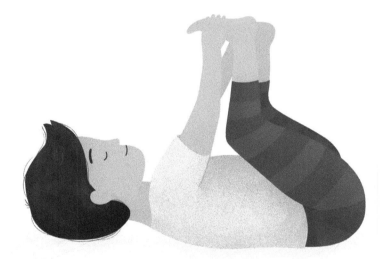

BOAT

ALL AGES

 STRENGTHENING

 CORE ENGAGING

Boat pose is a great introduction to core-strengthening poses, as the support of the ground makes it accessible and fun. Boat also presents lots of opportunities for fun engagement: ask kids to take a boat ride with you or sing "Row, Row, Row Your Boat" while holding the pose for longer increments of time. Try Boat whenever you need to re-energize and refresh.

1. Start in a seated position with your legs straight out in front of you.

2. Bend your knees toward you and set the soles of the feet on the ground in front of your bottom.

3. Place your hands behind your knees, engage the core muscles, and lift your feet off the ground so your calves and shins are parallel to the ground.

4. Take a deep breath. For more core engagement, reach your arms along your sides, palms facing one another.

5. Relax your shoulders by gently drawing the shoulder blades down the back.

6. For even more of a challenge, you can reach the legs straight up and away from you, forming a seated "V" shape with the body.

7. Breathe deeply a few times.

8. To release, set your feet back on the ground.

TIP

- While engaging the core in Boat, liven it up with a few snaps and claps as you breathe deeply. This focuses the mind and may help you and your kids hold this challenging pose a little longer.

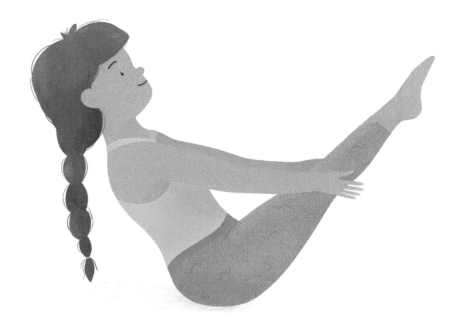

HERO

6 AND UP

 GROUNDING

 CALMING

This is a unique pose, as it invites us to feel grounded and supported while also stretching the calves, hips, and even the feet. Seated meditation and most breathing exercises can be done in Hero pose. This pose also improves posture and increases circulation in the lower body. Encourage your entire family to feel more confident and "like a hero" in this pose.

1. Start in Candle (page 74), and place a rolled blanket or towel between your calves and thighs if you need extra lift and support.

2. Sit back either onto the blanket or the ground between the legs, pressing the tops of the feet into the ground.

3. Take a deep breath in and elongate the spine.

4. Exhale and place the palms face-down on the tops of the thighs.

5. If your bottom doesn't reach the floor, place a block or stack of books underneath it for additional support.

6. Relax your shoulders by gently drawing the shoulder blades down the back.

7. Stay still as long as feels comfortable, taking deep breaths for 30 seconds to a few minutes.

8. To release, bring your hands by your sides, lift your torso, and swing the legs around so they are straight out in front of you.

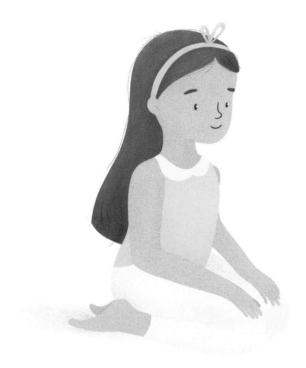

WIDE-LEGGED SEATED FORWARD BEND

ALL AGES

 GROUNDING

 CALMING

This grounding pose resembles the shape of a pizza slice (see tip). Connect to your breath as you stretch the groin and hips in this forward fold. Sit up on a folded blanket, bolster, or even a pillow to give the hips some lift and gain relief from the intensity of the groin stretch.

1. Start seated on the mat with your legs straight out in front of you. It may be helpful to sit up on a folded blanket.

2. Reach your legs out to the sides of the room as far as feels comfortable.

3. Inhale and place your fingertips behind the lower back, elongating through the spine.

4. Exhale and shift the hips back and the upper body forward, moving the fingertips in front of the pelvis and leaning forward into the fold.

5. Relax your shoulders by gently drawing the shoulder blades down the back.

6. Breathe deeply a few times, crawling your fingers out in front of you and folding deeper without pushing yourself or forcing a deeper fold.

7. Breathe into any aches and pains in the inner groin and back off the pose if it feels too intense.

8. Hold for a few deep breaths, growing long on the inhale and melting into the fold on the exhale.

9. To release, slowly return to a seated position.

TIP

• Make a pizza in this pose. With the legs wide and in the shape of a pizza slice, you can sprinkle cheese up and down the middle of the pose as you stretch, throw on some veggies, and use your creativity as you create your own personal pizza. Allow your child to lead this pose and only offer suggestions for the pizza toppings if she is reluctant to engage.

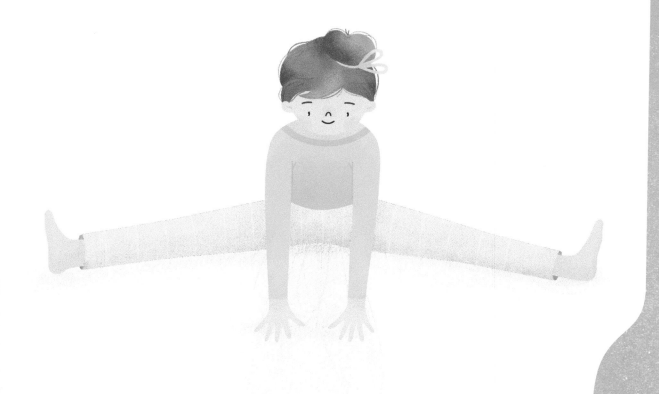

CRISS-CROSS

ALL AGES

 GROUNDING

 CALMING

Criss-Cross is the most common pose for seated meditation and generally the easiest pose in which to practice most breathing exercises. Most kids already know how to sit in Criss-Cross from other activities or school, so this is a great way to begin a yoga practice without a great deal of instruction involved.

1. Start seated on the mat with your legs straight out in front of you. It may be helpful to sit up on a folded blanket so your hips are higher than your knees.

2. Draw each foot in to tuck in under the opposite knee.

3. Take a deep inhale, and on the exhale, shift the hips back and tilt the pelvis slightly forward.

4. Elongate the spine as you take a few deep breaths.

5. Relax your shoulders by gently drawing the shoulder blades down the back.

6. Allow your gaze to be soft.

7. Hold for a few deep breaths.

TIP

- In Criss-Cross, ask kids to "follow me" and create a rhythm by tapping your legs, snapping, and clapping. Lift your arms overhead with an inhale, press the palms together, and take a big exhale as you pull the palms to the heart. Create any interesting rhythm or movement (you can even make a silly face) for them to imitate and to add a fun energy to your practice.

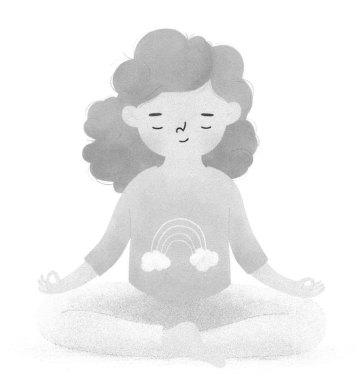

LOTUS

ALL AGES

 GROUNDING

 CALMING

An advanced seated pose, Lotus may come only after many years of practice. Don't let this deter you from trying it out periodically. The pose feels good and grounding regardless of your ability level. And be warned, many little ones are more flexible than their adult counterparts and can do this pose easily! Once you can comfortably sit in this pose, try it during a meditation exercise or to unwind at the beginning of a yoga session.

1. Start in a seated position with your legs straight out in front of you.

2. Inhale and bend one knee, pressing the foot into the ground. Bring the opposite knee up into a cradle with your arms.

3. Exhale and set the cradled foot down in the crook of the opposite thigh near the hip. If at any point you feel pain in the knee, take a deep, slow breath and gently release the pose.

4. Breathing deeply, take the other foot and gently set it down on top of the leg in the crook of the thigh near the hip.

5. Relax your shoulders by gently drawing the shoulder blades down the back, elongating the spine.

6. Take your hands and rest them softly on the legs.

7. Breathe into any tightness.

8. To release the pose, slowly release the top leg and move into a comfortable seated position.

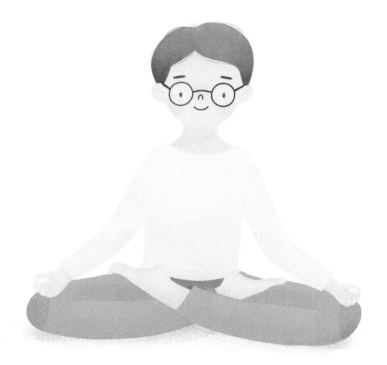

SEATED FIGURE "4"

ALL AGES

 GROUNDING

 CALMING

This pose is a wonderful way to open the hips while feeling the support of the ground beneath you. It also helps relieve lower back tension. Try this right off the bat with younger kids, because they love to make number shapes with their bodies. Regardless of age, using the number "4" as an instructional cue helps the practitioner gain easier access to the position.

1. Sit down with your feet planted on the ground and the knees bent.

2. Place your hands by your sides.

3. Cross your right ankle over the left thigh, creating a number "4" shape with the legs.

4. Elongate the spine and relax the neck and shoulders.

5. Gently lift up and shift your torso closer toward the right heel.

6. Pause and take a few deep breaths.

7. Release the right leg and pause for a moment with both legs stretched in front of you.

8. Repeat on the other side.

TIP

- Make this pose more active by engaging the core and lifting your bottom off the ground on an exhale, and then lowering on the inhale. Repeat 10 times.

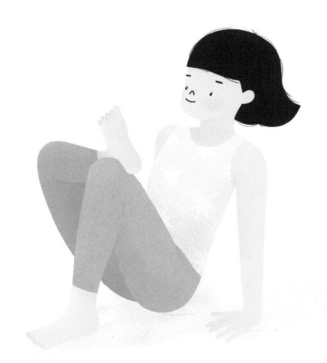

CHAPTER

7

BENDS
& TWISTS

Bends and twists provide for a well-rounded yoga practice. Kids enjoy the physical challenge of both bends and twists. Twisting poses are a way to energize the body and release lower-back tension. Twists are a great way to introduce kids to the concept of body awareness and balance, as they require focus on the sides of the body as well as the body as a whole. Twists can even provide a framework for little ones to understand the left and right sides of their bodies. Forward folds cultivate calm and ground feelings. Use forward folds when you or your child need a moment to release tension or unwind from a long day. Forward folds may feel a bit creaky at first in the lower back and knees—don't be afraid to bend the knees and assist your body in the way it needs as you practice forward folds. Backbends tend to energize and invigorate the body. They help release tension and open the chest and heart area of the body. Gentle backbends are a therapeutic way to relieve tension at the end of a long day, while Wheel (page 124) and Bow (page 126) can set the tone for an energetic outlook in the morning.

RECLINED TWIST

ALL AGES

 GROUNDING

 CALMING

This is a nurturing twist that's easy for everyone. It's a popular closing pose to use before your final resting pose and relaxation. It also feels great after Happy Baby (page 92). You can hold the twist on each side for as long as feels comfortable.

1. Start by lying on your back.

2. Draw your knees into your chest.

3. Keeping your knees in at your chest, reach your arms out to both sides.

4. Inhale and imagine every part of your body touching the ground getting heavier and softer.

5. Exhale and allow the legs to drop to the right side. Gaze over your left shoulder to deepen the twist. Take a few deep breaths.

6. To release, draw the knees back into the chest.

7. Repeat on the other side.

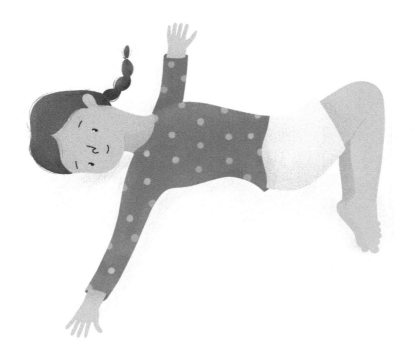

WIDE-LEGGED FORWARD FOLD

ALL AGES

 GROUNDING

 CALMING

This forward fold is a great way to release the spine while stretching the inner thighs. The pose releases tension and soothes the nervous system. You can signal alignment to kids by showing them how this pose creates a triangle shape with their bodies. If the feet are too close together, the pose can feel inaccessible. Help everybody find the right width in the feet before setting up the pose.

1. Start in Star (page 64) and place your hands on your hips.

2. Take a slight bend in your knees, and gradually straighten the legs.

3. Take a deep breath and grow longer through your spine.

4. Fold the torso and arms forward toward the floor, hinging at the hips and keeping your spine long. When you're as low as feels comfortable, let your palms rest on the floor. Use a block or stack of books under your hands if you can't comfortably reach the floor.

5. Allow your neck and shoulders to relax into gravity.

6. Breathe deeply a few times.

7. To release, engage the core, place your hands on your hips, and lift up to standing while keeping the spine long.

TIPS

- Turn this into a shoulder opener by grabbing your opposite elbows or clasping the hands behind your back.
- Add in taps on the floor, snap one hand at a time while folded down, or sway from side to side to create a more active pose for wiggly bodies.

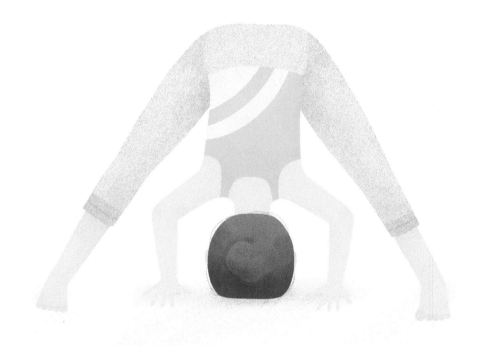

PUPPY

ALL AGES

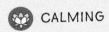 CALMING

Puppy is a soothing hybrid between Down Dog (page 52) and Child's Pose (page 46). Many younger children love this pose simply because of the cute name and very puppy-like position. It is also a wonderful stretch for adults, as it extends the spine while opening the shoulders and heart region. Try this pose together as a family after a long car or airplane ride.

1. Start in Candle (page 74) and then sit back on your heels.

2. Walk your hands forward and reach your arms toward the top of the mat. Press the fingers and palms down as if you were doing Down Dog (page 52), and lift the hips and bottom toward the back of your mat.

3. Lengthen through the arms and the spine and rest your forehead on the mat.

4. Take slow, deep breaths. Feel the upper body engage and the shoulders and neck soften.

5. To release, slowly lift the upper body back into Candle and take a comfortable seated position.

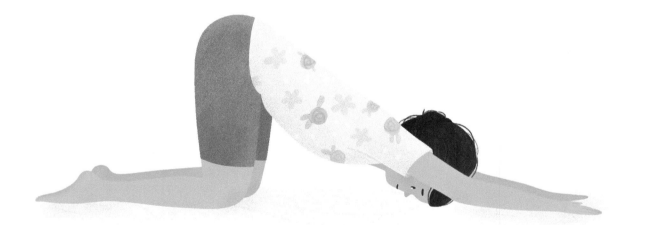

SEATED TWIST

ALL AGES

 GROUNDING

 CALMING

This pose is an easy way to counter long bouts of sitting still or inactivity. One way to feel a greater stretch in this pose is to elongate through the spine while making sure your neck and shoulders are relaxed. Simple and effective, this pose can also be done while in a chair, keeping your feet planted on the ground. Try this as a break during screen time: stop what you're doing to hit "pause" and take a few twists and breaths as a way to reconnect with your body and mind.

1. Start in Criss-Cross (page 100).
2. Reach both arms up and twist to the right side.
3. Put the left hand on the right knee as you twist, and place the right hand on the ground behind you.
4. Take a deep inhale and elongate the spine. Exhale, and twist a little deeper using the hand on the knee to help deepen the twist.
5. Relax your shoulders and neck, drawing the shoulder blades down the back.
6. Release the pose and take a few deep breaths.
7. Repeat on the other side.

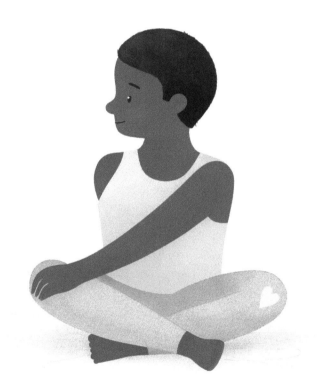

LOW LUNGE TWIST

ALL AGES

 GROUNDING

 CALMING

Low Lunge Twist provides the stability of the knee on the ground while you turn and twist. This is a great way to refresh and renew while stretching the lower back. This twist can be done quickly and efficiently while providing great benefit. Try holding the twist for longer periods of time while connecting to the breath and gaining access to a deep stretch in the quadriceps and hips.

1. Start in Down Dog (page 52).

2. Step your right foot forward to the top of the mat, keeping some space between the feet so the hips have room to twist.

3. Set your left knee down to the mat and untuck your toes.

4. Reach both arms up with the palms facing each other, shoulders relaxing down the back.

5. Twist your torso to the right, twisting from the core and gazing back behind you.

6. To go a little deeper, drop the left elbow outside of the right knee and draw the palms together, pressing them against your sternum. Inhale and elongate the spine. On the exhale, twist deeper into the pose.

7. Release the twist and rest your hands on your right thigh for a few breaths.

8. Repeat on the second side.

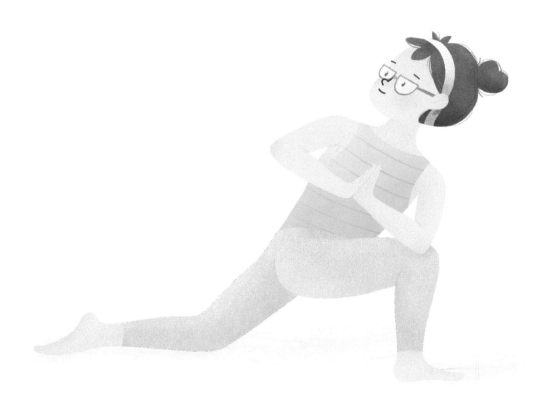

TWISTING TRIANGLE

7 AND UP

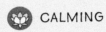 CALMING

Twisting Triangle demands our focus and challenges us to be steady in our legs and breath. This is a more challenging pose to build up to as your yoga practice progresses. The position can feel a little confusing in the beginning, but remember to keep a sense of humor and play around with it. Use a block or a stack of books against the outside of the bottom foot to gain access to the pose if needed. This pose promotes focus, flexibility, and patience, along with a growth mind-set.

1. Start in Triangle (page 70) with the right leg forward, and shorten the stance between your legs.

2. Breathing in, reach the left arm forward and send the hips toward the back of the mat, gently bending your knees.

3. Place your left hand on the outside of your right foot, by the pinky toe. Use a block or stack of books if you need additional support.

4. Rotate the hips and twist to the right, reaching your right arm up to the sky.

5. Gaze up at your right hand, relaxing the neck. If you feel any pain in the neck, look down at the ground.

6. To release, engage the core and lift the torso and chest back up. Place the left foot next to the right in Mountain (page 40).

7. Repeat on the other side.

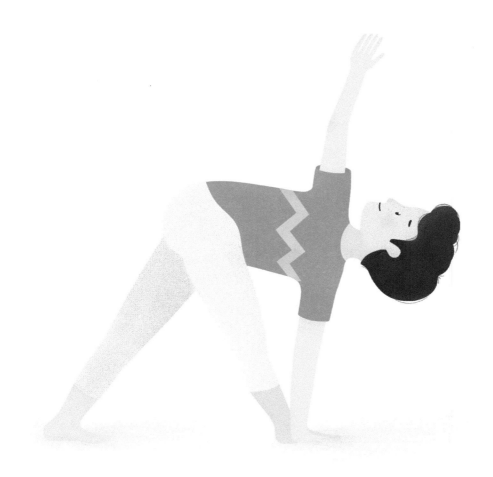

UP DOG

ALL AGES

 REJUVENATING

Up Dog presents another fun opportunity for young kids to imitate animals while growing their yoga practice. It is a rejuvenating backbend, and slightly more intense than Cobra (page 58). The key here is to press your hands and the tops of your feet into the ground while lifting everything else. The pose will make you feel light and elevated and is a great heart opener.

1. Start by lying facedown on your mat.

2. Stretch your legs straight behind you with the tops of your feet pressing into the floor.

3. Place your palms on the ground a few inches behind your armpits, next to the rib cage. Bend your elbows so they point straight back (not out to the sides).

4. Inhale and press the hands down even more as you move the torso and hips forward and up. Lift the body through Cobra (page 58), and then lift the thighs and shins off the floor, pressing firmly into the tops of your feet.

5. Exhale and relax your neck as you engage the legs and draw the shoulder blades slightly down the back. Gaze up toward the sky, and take a few deep breaths.

6. To release, lower your legs, torso, and head gently back down to the floor.

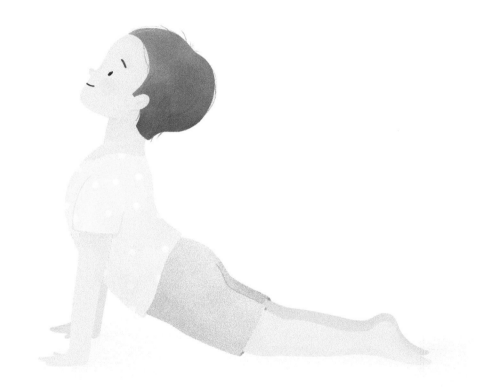

CAMEL

4 AND UP

 ENERGIZING

This pose builds energy and increases flexibility in the spine. Camel feels wonderful when the shoulder and heart areas are tight. It's important to move slowly and carefully in this pose to protect the lower back. This pose provides similar benefits to Wheel (page 124), while offering more stability with the knees planted on the ground. Pay attention to the way your neck feels in this pose. You can keep a slight tuck of the chin in order to protect the neck if necessary. As you breathe through this pose, enjoy the opening in the heart, neck and shoulders.

1. Start in Candle (page 74). For added lift, tuck the toes under and lift the heels. For a deeper stretch, allow the tops of the feet to remain on the floor.

2. Place your hands on your hips and then rotate the elbows so they point to the back of your mat behind you. The hands may also rotate to the back of the hips and pelvis.

3. Engage the core and allow the hips to press forward slightly as you lift up and back through the torso and chest.

4. Press into your hands and lift the chest, gently drawing the shoulder blades down the back, and letting the head and neck relax as you arch backward.

5. If you feel steady, you may reach your hands back and down to grab your heels. Otherwise, keep your hands at your hips.

6. Take a few deep breaths.

7. To release, engage the core and take the hands back to the hips. Slowly lift the body into Candle, allowing the neck and head to come up last.

8. Counterbalance this pose by stretching in Puppy (page 112) or Child's Pose (page 46).

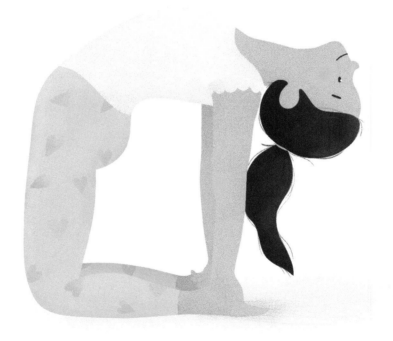

WHEEL

5 AND UP

 ENERGIZING

This is a challenging backbend with invigorating results. It's a favorite with young gymnasts and dancers. In Wheel, your perspective is visually shifted upside down and you gain access to a vigorous heart opener. Kids naturally gravitate toward this pose and yearn to achieve it, as it looks fun. It's important to remind your child (and yourself!) to breathe through this pose and that achieving the pose in its full form is really not the end goal. This is a great pose for teaching patience and a growth mind-set.

1. Start by lying on your back.

2. Bend your knees and draw your feet in toward your bottom.

3. Reach your hands up toward the ceiling and over your head. Place your hands down by the ears, palms down and fingers pointing toward the feet.

4. Inhale and relax the body.

5. Exhale and press the hands and feet down firmly. Engage the core, and raise your hips and chest up off the ground, pressing as high as you can.

6. Allow your head to hang back, and relax the neck. Take a few deep breaths.

7. To release, lower the hips and tuck your chin into the chest as you slowly lower your spine to the ground.

8. Place your hands on the belly and keep your knees bent up toward the ceiling for a few gentle breaths.

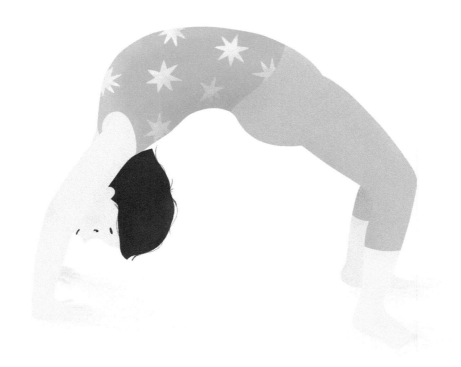

BOW

4 AND UP

 ENERGIZING

Bow pose is a backbend with the unique aspect of the belly pressing on the ground as the back arches in the shape of a bow. Bow opens the heart and aids the digestive system. Be careful not to practice this pose on a full stomach, as it may feel quite uncomfortable! Bow is also a great pose to ignite the imagination and create a simple yoga story for those kids who like an adventure. Aim your bow toward your wishes and goals and imagine them landing smoothly (and safely!) within sight.

1. Lie facedown on the mat with your legs straight out behind you.

2. Draw your feet in toward your bottom and take a big inhale.

3. Exhale and lift the torso and chest as you reach back with your hands to grab the outer edges of your feet.

4. Inhale and then exhale and press your feet into your hands and raise your thighs off the ground, arching back toward your feet. Allow the belly to feel soft and relax your eyes, gazing straight ahead. Take a few breaths here.

5. Relax your shoulders by gently drawing the shoulder blades down the back.

6. To release, lower the legs, release the feet, and gently lower the upper body and legs to the ground.

TIP

- Turn your bow on its side and rock and roll with bow pose. Kids love to roll around while keeping their legs and arms in bow pose.

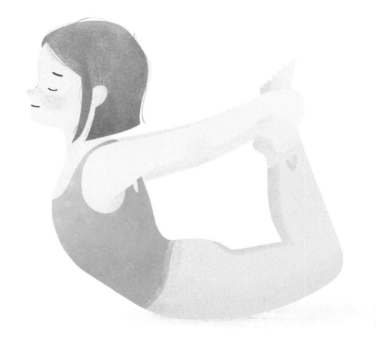

STANDING SPLITS

7 AND UP

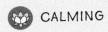 CALMING

Standing Splits is a fun and satisfying challenge. Remember that it doesn't matter how high the back leg lifts—the important thing is to keep the back hip square to the ground and breathe as you find your balance. If you realize you've stopped breathing, readjust! Flexible little ones may have an easier time with this pose than adults. Just go at your own pace and encourage each other to have fun while wobbling in this pose.

1. Start in Mountain (page 40).

2. Take a deep inhale, and as you exhale, move into Forward Fold (page 42). Be mindful not to lock your knees; a slight bend in the knees keeps them safe from injury.

3. Take a deep inhale and reach your hands slightly forward. If the floor feels too far away, use blocks or a stack of books under the hands. Shift your weight onto your right foot.

4. As you exhale, reach the left leg up behind you. Keep the leg and hip pointing toward the floor as you continue to lift the leg.

5. Take a few deep breaths and relax the neck and shoulders, keeping your left leg active and pressing away from you.

6. If you feel steady and confident, walk your hands back closer toward your right foot.

7. Breathe deeply a few times.

8. To release, gently lower the lifted leg and place it next to your standing foot. Take a breath in Forward Fold before rising to stand.

9. Repeat on the other side.

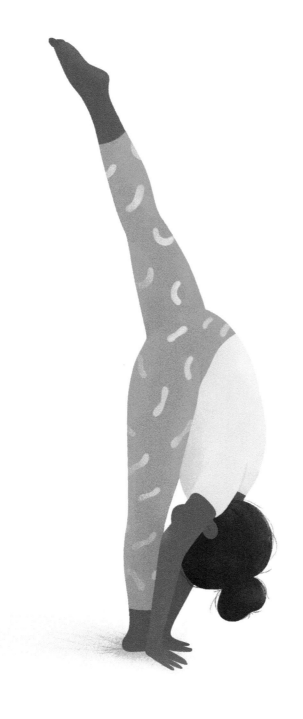

HIGH LUNGE TWIST

5 AND UP

 GROUNDING

 CALMING

High Lunge Twist strengthens the legs while engaging the core, hips, and shoulders. When teaching younger children to "engage the core," you can simply say "Feel your belly, and while you breathe, make it really strong." It's important not to give too many instructions that might cause kids to become unnecessarily tense. This powerful twist is a fun challenge to build focus and balance.

1. Start in a High Lunge (page 80) with your right foot forward.

2. Set your left hand down on the inside of the right foot. You can place a block or stack of books under the hand for added support.

3. Inhale and lengthen the right arm up toward the sky, then exhale, twisting toward the right.

4. Relax your shoulders by gently drawing the shoulder blades down the back, and elongate the spine.

5. Breathe deeply a few times, feeling length through the torso and arms and stability in the lower body.

6. Release the twist and come back to High Lunge. Repeat on the other side.

TIP

- To build in more fun for kids in this pose, release the hand from the floor and lift the torso up while maintaining a twist. Reach the arms wide and add a few snaps. Pivot the back foot to a 45-degree angle, reaching the arms wide in Warrior 2 (page 68) on the opposite side. Make a couple of snaps here. Then turn on the ball of the foot, lift back into the twist with the torso lifted, and make a couple of snaps with the arms extended. This is a great way to add rhythm and balance to the pose.

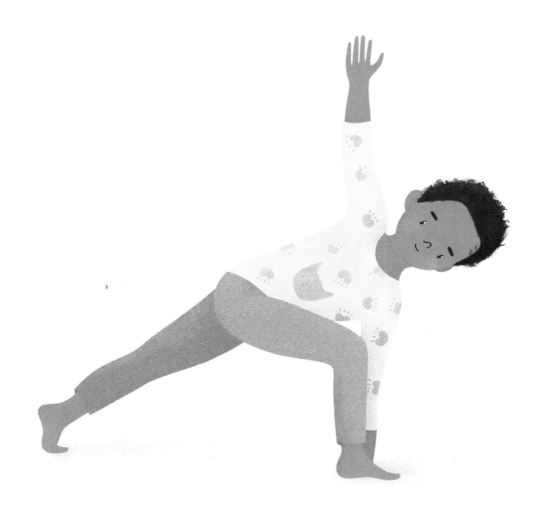

CHAPTER

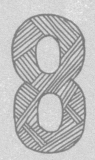

8

BALANCE

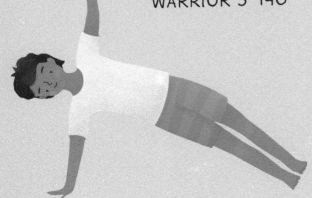

Balancing poses are popular with kids, as they love the physical challenge of standing on one leg or even one hand and one foot (see how much they like Side Plank, page 144!). The focus point of the eyes while in balancing poses can make a big difference in how the pose feels. When you learn to keep your eyes glued to one spot while holding a balancing pose, you engage the mind-body connection. It's amazing how quickly these poses can quiet the mind. And remember, wobbling and falling is totally okay! If your child begins falling on purpose or exaggerating her fall, use inquiry and show her how to fall safely. As a general rule of thumb, once we give kids permission to fall, their desire to fall for the sake of silliness is less alluring. Build focus and relieve stress by breathing through the challenges of balancing poses. Encourage your child to feel stable, grounded, patient, and confident as they explore these poses.

TREE

ALL AGES

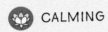 CALMING

Tree is a wonderful pose to introduce the concept of balance and stability. As we balance on one leg, we experiment with different placements of our raised leg and arms. Tree pose also stokes the imagination as you can "become" any type of tree or take an adventure to the forest as you practice the pose.

1. Start in Mountain (page 40).

2. Shift your weight onto your left leg and find a focal point for the eyes in front of you on the ground.

3. Turn your right knee out to the right side of the room.

4. Lift your right heel above the left ankle, pressing the heel into the inside of the left shin.

5. Press your palms together at your sternum and take a breath.

6. Reach your palms straight up overhead as you press firmly into the left foot.

7. If you feel steady, lift the right foot higher on the shin, being careful not to press the foot against the knee.

8. For an extra challenge, draw the right foot all the way up to the inner left thigh. Breathe deeply a few times.

9. To release, set the right foot down next to the left.

10. Repeat on the other side.

TIP

• Have fun with it! Reach both arms up and blow your branches in the wind.

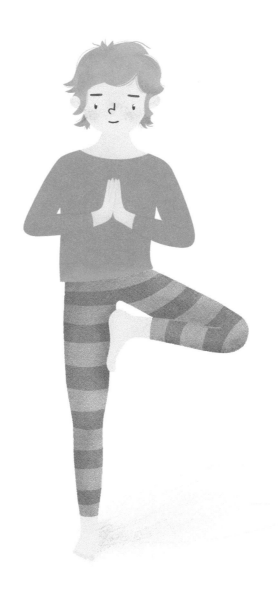

EAGLE

7 AND UP

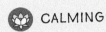 CALMING

Get ready to take flight with Eagle pose! Build confidence and stability as you practice your connection to your breath. Eagle pose steadies the mind while opening the hips and improving balance. Remind your family that falling out of this pose is okay! Steady yourself by setting both feet down and trying again, connecting to your breath and playful attitude.

1. Start in Mountain (page 40).

2. Bend your knees and then take your right knee over your left, squeezing your inner thighs together. Lower your bottom toward the ground, balancing on your left foot. If that feels unsteady, bend the right knee and cross your right ankle over the left knee, making a "4." Take a few breaths.

3. Inhale and lift the arms. Cross your left elbow under your right elbow and bring your palms together. Exhale and press your forearms away from your face, feeling the stretch between your shoulder blades. Take a few deep breaths.

4. To release, uncross the arms and place your right knee down by your left.

5. Repeat on the other side.

TIP

- Try Eagle on your back first. This helps the body understand the position with support from the ground. This is great for kids who feel the need to perfect a pose and have trouble trying it if it seems too challenging. You can also add rhythm by lifting the arms up (still pressing them together) on the inhale and pulling them back down on the exhale.

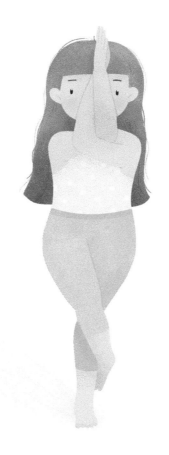

DANCER

ALL AGES

 REJUVENATING

Dancer is both a balancing pose and a backbend. Little ones will have fun pretending they are a ballet dancer or ice skater while holding this pretty pose. If at any point you feel like you will fall out of the pose, simply place your foot on the floor and try again. You can also do this pose with your back foot against a wall for added support.

1. Start in Mountain (page 40).

2. Inhale and shift your weight onto your right foot, lifting your left heel up and toward your bottom.

3. Exhale and reach the left arm back to grab the outside of your left foot.

4. Breathe deeply, and find a spot on the ground in front of you to focus your gaze, keeping it steady and soft.

5. Inhale again and press the left foot into the left hand. Use a towel or strap to grab the back foot if you have tight hamstrings and can't quite reach your foot with your hand.

6. Reach the right arm straight in front of you, parallel to the floor.

7. Take a few deep breaths.

8. To release, lower the left foot next to the right.

9. Repeat on the other side.

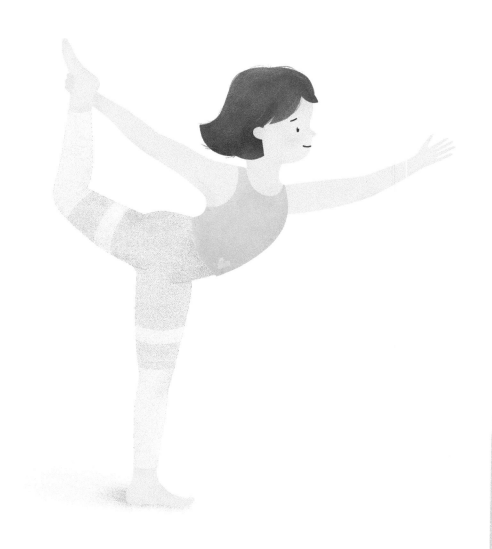

WARRIOR 3

5 AND UP

 REJUVENATING

Warrior 3 is also known as "Fierce Warrior." While this balancing pose is challenging, it also requires a sense of calm and ease and a steadiness in the breath. The key is rooting down through the standing leg and keeping your back leg strong and active. Remind kids that a true warrior is strong yet calm. You may want to practice this pose against a wall, pressing the back foot into the wall for additional support.

1. Start in Warrior 2 (page 68) with the right foot forward.

2. Press into the toes and ball of the left foot, turning the heel up toward the ceiling.

3. Inhale and lean your weight onto the right foot as you lift your left foot off the ground and left leg into the air parallel to the ground.

4. Reach the arms forward, palms facing each other, as the leg lifts and the back foot presses back as if into a wall. Exhale.

5. Find your focal point on the ground in front of you.

6. Spend a few rounds of breath here, building focus and stability.

7. To release, simply set the foot down.

8. Repeat on the other side.

TIP

- Turn Warrior 3 into a fun airplane ride, asking your child where she wants to go. As you hold the pose, explain what you see on the way. When you release the pose, pretend you're landing at the airport. My daughter often asks to go to New York and we marvel at the Rocky Mountains along the way, making sure to land at JFK and grab a burger in the terminal at the end.

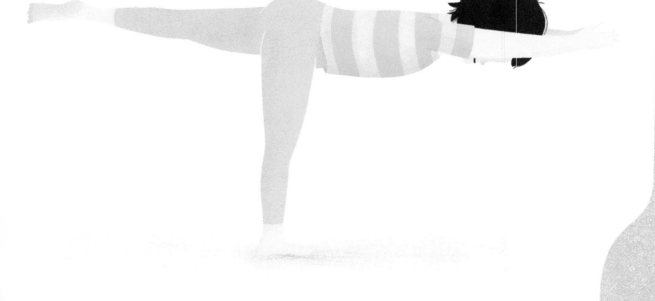

HALF MOON

5 AND UP

 REJUVENATING

Half Moon is another challenging balancing pose that also opens up the side body. The big difference with Half Moon compared to Warrior 3 (page 140) or Standing Splits (page 128) is that the hips are open to the side, rather than square with the ground. You can practice this pose against a wall with the back foot pressing into the wall for additional support.

1. Start in Side Angle (page 78) with the right foot forward at the front of the mat.

2. Gaze at a point in front of the right knee and lean your weight forward, lifting your right arm off your thigh.

3. Inhale and press into the left foot and then lift it off the ground parallel to the floor, hips open to the side, and simultaneously place the right hand underneath the right shoulder. Place the right hand on a block or a stack of books if you need added support. Keep your gaze to the side of the room, and raise your left arm up toward the sky.

4. Exhale and lengthen through the back leg and through both arms. Relax your shoulders by gently drawing the shoulder blades down the back. Take a few deep breaths.

5. To release, gently set the left foot back on the ground.

6. Repeat on the other side.

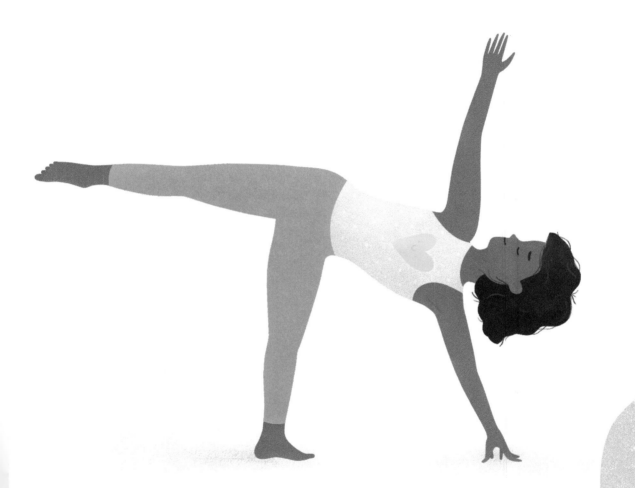

SIDE PLANK

5 AND UP

 ENERGIZING

 STRENGTHENING

Side Plank is an arm balance and also improves strength in the upper and lower body. If you're still building your strength, place your lower knee down for added support during this pose. Over time, you'll be able to hold the pose for longer increments on both sides. This is a challenging pose, so remember to breathe and have fun!

1. Begin in Plank (page 54).

2. Take a deep inhale and shift your weight onto your right hand, rolling onto the outer edge of your right foot.

3. Press the feet together and reach the left arm up, making a straight line with the right arm. Keep your hip high and press the right hand firmly into the ground.

4. Exhale and hold your gaze steady toward the side of the room. Keep your core engaged and your neck and face relaxed. Continue reaching up with your left arm to get some lift in the pose. Take a few deep breaths.

5. To release, return to Plank.

6. Repeat on the other side.

TIP

- Try playing Follow Me (page 170) with snaps, waves, and silly sounds while in this pose. Ask children to notice whether maintaining a sense of humor throughout the pose helps take the focus off the challenge in the arms.

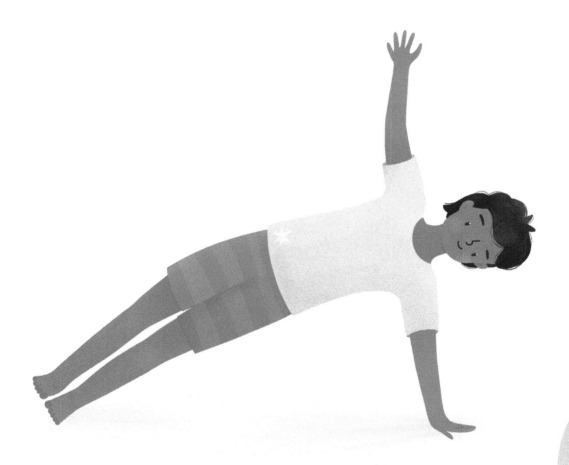

CROW

5 AND UP

 ENERGIZING

 STRENGTHENING

Children love the physical challenge of the arm-balancing Crow pose. Adults tend to find it a bit more challenging and intimidating. This pose is a wonderful opportunity to both model and teach a growth mind-set, as it can take many months (or years!) to get into Crow. This pose improves balance, builds arm strength, and relies on an efficient distribution of weight in the body.

1. Begin in Frog (page 82).

2. Reach your arms down to the ground and lower your shoulders down to the insides of your knees.

3. Press your hands firmly into the ground. Settle your gaze on a spot just in front of your hands and hold your gaze during Crow.

4. Inhale and lift onto the balls of your feet, then exhale, bend your elbows, and press your shins into the back of your upper arms.

5. Engage your core and try lifting one foot off the ground. Return it to the ground and try lifting the other foot.

6. Take a big inhale and on the exhale, keeping the core engaged, lift both feet off the ground, resting the knees against the backs of your arms as if they're on a little shelf. Lean your head forward toward your gaze to help distribute some of your weight forward.

7. Focus on your inhale and exhale. Breathe deeply a few times to stabilize the pose.

8. Release the feet down to the ground.

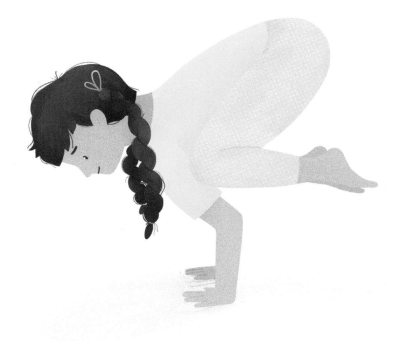

HANDSTAND VARIATION

7 AND UP

 ENERGIZING

 STRENGTHENING

This fun inversion pose requires a sense of humor, a growth mind-set, and concentration all at once. It's a great way to get moving and appeals to those who love a challenge. Kids will have fun watching adults try this upside-down position. You might be surprised to see them tracking your progress in the pose as closely as they track their own. Handstand Variation is a fun, safe way to feel stability in an arm balance and slowly build up to a handstand.

1. Place your yoga mat against a wall with plenty of space around you in all directions.

2. Start in Table Top (page 44) with the bottom of your feet pressing against the wall.

3. Gradually walk the legs up the wall so that your hips are at a 90-degree angle and your body forms an "L" shape.

4. Keep your gaze just in front of your hands and breathe into the neck to soften it, even as the rest of the body is working hard. Make sure your shoulders are directly over your wrists.

5. Press the hands firmly into the ground and press the right foot into the wall.

6. Engage the core muscles and lift the left leg straight up toward the ceiling.

7. If you feel steady, practice pressing the right foot into the wall even more for leverage and lift it up to meet the left leg. Keep the shoulders strong and breathe deeply.

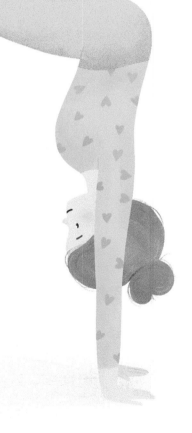

8. To release, bring the legs down to the ground safely and move into Down Dog (page 52) or Child's Pose (page 46).

9. Repeat, lifting the right foot up first. Ask kids to notice any difference in the pose or preference for sides.

CHAPTER

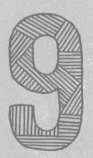

9

PARTNER POSES

Partner poses are a great way to build fun into your yoga routine at home or on the go. Kids love partner poses because they are interactive and leave more room for connecting and giggling during yoga. Partner poses are a simple way to build focus, teamwork, and empathy. Use partner poses to practice other nonverbal skills like eye contact (when possible) and nodding. Be sure to demonstrate a sense of humor as you get into the partner poses so everyone knows it's okay to laugh and be silly. Just remind kids to breathe and concentrate so no one gets hurt.

For three-year olds, it's best to practice all the partner poses with an adult. Children ages four and up can practice these poses with a sibling or friend, or an adult.

DOUBLE DOG

ALL AGES

 REJUVENATING

Double Dog is as simple and fun as it sounds. It's basically two people stacking Down Dog. The first gets into the pose, and the second uses the other person's lower back as the ground as they get into the pose next. This is a great pose to teach teamwork and communication. Ask kids to switch off who gets to be "top dog," and let them have fun rubbing each other's backs with their feet.

1. Partner A (grown-up) starts in Down Dog (page 52).

2. Partner B starts in Forward Fold (page 42) with her heels directly in front of Partner A's fingertips.

3. Partner B carefully walks her feet up Partner A's back, adjusting her hands on the ground as necessary.

4. Partner B places each foot on the side of Partner A's lower back, and gently presses into Partner A's back with her feet.

5. Both partners hold the pose for a few rounds of breath.

6. To release, Partner B walks her hands forward to gain clearance for her feet, and gently places her feet down on the outside of Partner A's hands.

7. Switch roles if everybody feels safe.

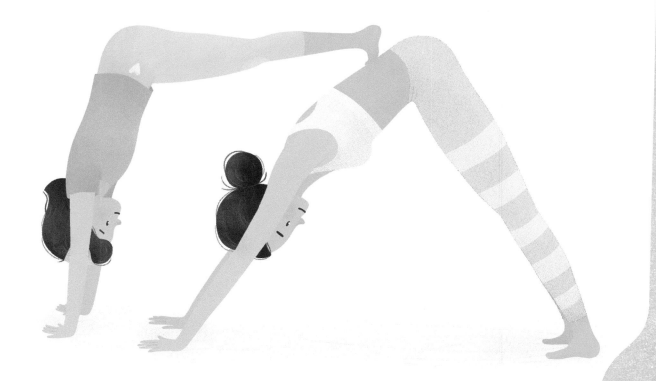

BACK-TO-BACK CHAIR

ALL AGES

 REJUVENATING

This pose requires strong communication skills and engages kids with a fun challenge to lift off the ground. Both partners will build core strength and balance. Tuning into the position of the other person also promotes empathy, connection, and listening.

1. Partner A and Partner B sit on the floor, back-to-back.

2. Both partners bend their knees up toward the ceiling and link elbows behind them.

3. Being careful to distribute body weight appropriately (grown-ups may ask little ones to lean back with more force), both partners press into each other's backs and press their feet down into the floor.

4. Partner A and Partner B lift up together into Chair (page 72), keeping their elbows linked.

5. Partners hold the pose, taking a few deep breaths. When ready, they decide to lower down together.

6. To release the pose, both partners use their leg muscles to slowly guide each other down to the ground and back into a seated position.

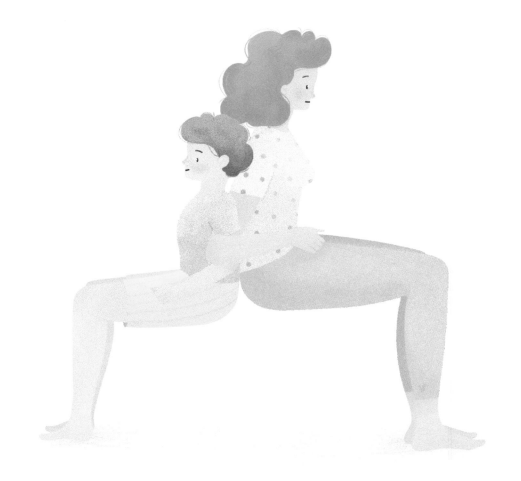

DOUBLE TREE

ALL AGES

 REJUVENATING

Double Tree is a simple partner pose for grown-ups and children of all ages that improves balance and encourages eye contact (if possible). Kids can easily do this one together and will have fun pretending to be various kinds of trees in different places.

1. Start in Tree (page 134), facing each other.

2. Mirror your poses so Partner A is balancing on the right leg and Partner B is balancing on the left leg.

3. Partners raise their arms and press their hands together at the top of the tree. (If one partner is significantly taller, they can simply meet the hands of the smaller person.)

4. Take a few deep breaths and make eye contact as you both stand tall in your Tree.

5. To release, both partners set their elevated foot down next to the standing foot and lower their arms.

6. Repeat on the other side.

ACTIVITY

- Try waving your "branches" in the wind while holding the pose. Call out different places and weather patterns for your tree.

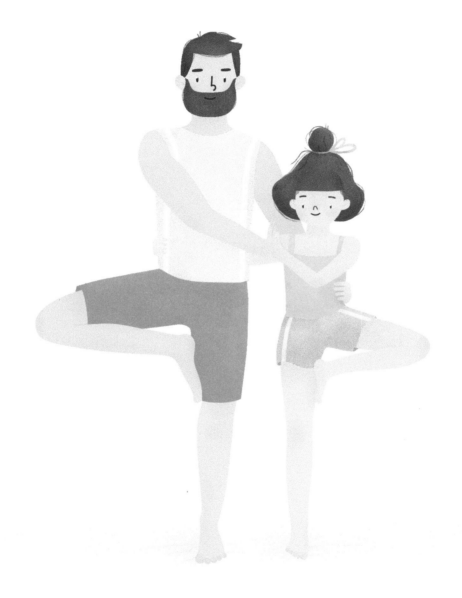

PARTNER SEATED TWIST

ALL AGES

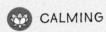 CALMING

This is a soothing, supported stretch through the upper body and an accessible partner pose that doesn't require any acrobatics or balance. If little ones are distracted, this is a great pose for kicking off partner work or your daily practice.

1. Both partners sit in Criss-Cross (page 100) facing one another with their knees touching.

2. Both people reach their right arm around their lower back.

3. Each reaches their left hand out to grab the other's right hand. If it's hard to reach hands, one partner can hold a towel and each person can grab one end of the towel.

4. Keep twisting together, possibly grabbing each other's wrists for a deeper stretch.

5. Repeat on the second side.

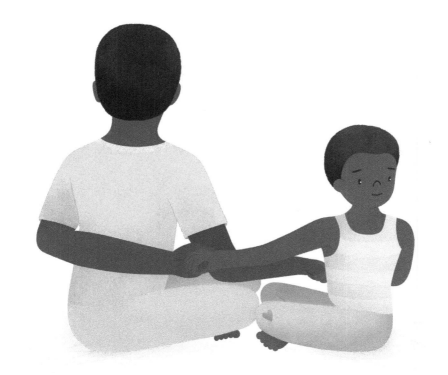

AIRPLANE

ALL AGES

 ENERGIZING

 STRENGTHENING

A classic! Enjoy this ride and allow your imaginations to soar. If this is done with an adult and child, the adult should be Partner A. Siblings and friends can also do this together, but if there is a big size difference, the bigger child should be Partner A. Take your little one on a ride to the park, a favorite playground, or even another country while improving their balance and body awareness.

1. Partner A lies with her back on the ground with knees bent and pointing toward the ceiling.

2. Partner B stands just in front of Partner A's knees.

3. Partner A gently presses her feet to Partner B's belly and takes hold of both of Partner B's hands.

4. As Partner B leans into Partner A, Partner A lifts Partner B with her feet, straightening her legs and maintaining a firm grasp with her hands.

5. Partner A flies Partner B in the air.

6. Switch positions if appropriate and safe.

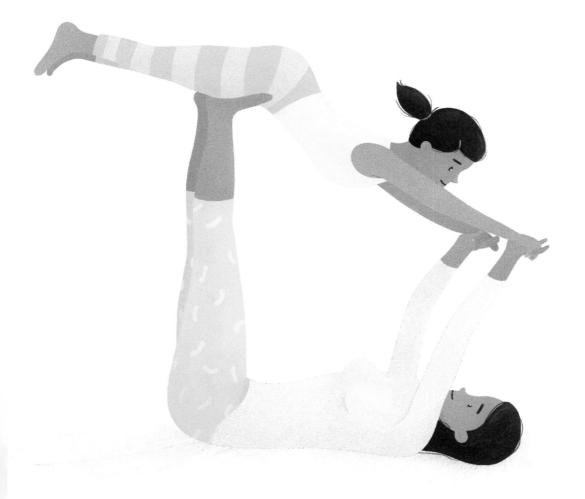

DOUBLE GATE

ALL AGES

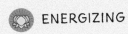 ENERGIZING

This is a great side stretch and a pose supported by gravity, with the standing knee on the ground providing a stable foundation.

1. Start in Candle (page 74) with both partners facing the same direction in a parallel line about 12 inches apart. Partner A starts with her left knee and leg on the interior side of the pose, and Partner B's right knee is on the inside of the pose.

2. Partner A extends her leg to the left, toward the middle of her mat and Partner B. Partner B reaches her leg to the right, toward the middle of the mat and Partner A.

3. Partner A reaches her right arm up and over her right ear toward Partner B's left extended arm, which is reaching up and over her left ear. This makes an arch or rainbow shape.

4. Both partners press their palms together or hold hands at the top of the arch and take a few deep breaths.

5. The partners can also hold hands with the bottom hand.

TIP

- Get creative and open and shut the gate. Release the top hand and lift the torso more upright to open the gate. To shut it, stretch back toward one another and press your palms together.

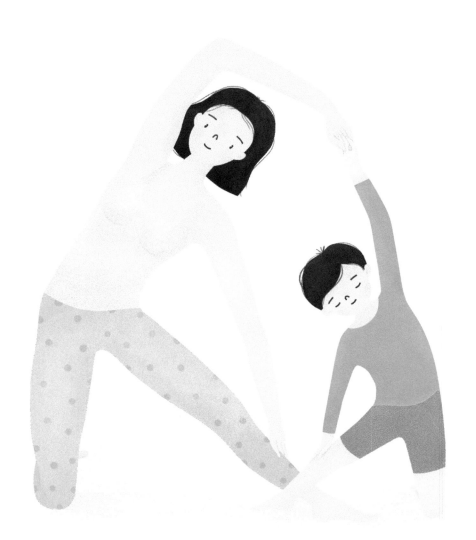

DOUBLE BOAT

ALL AGES

 ENERGIZING

 STRENGTHENING

Go on an aquatic adventure in Double Boat. This pose teaches teamwork and fires up the core to release energy. It also requires balance and knowing your limits. If there is a big size difference between the partners, straight legs might not be possible. Just take it as far as you can and have fun in the process.

1. Partners start by sitting on the ground facing each other. Each partner has their knees pulled in and up toward the ceiling and feet flat on the floor.

2. Partners press the soles of their feet into the other partner's feet, creating leverage in the legs. Partners can grab each other's hands for a deeper connection.

3. Continue pressing the feet together, keeping the knees bent, as each person lifts and lengthens through the spine.

4. As the partners maintain their connection in the hands and feet, they slowly begin to straighten their knees as far as is comfortable.

5. If straight knees aren't possible, partners can stay in the pose with their knees bent. As they hold the pose, partners take a few deep breaths together, maintaining eye contact and maybe even smiling.

6. To release, each partner lowers their feet to the ground and releases their hands.

TIP

- For those who love challenges, use a timer and build up the length of time you hold the pose together.

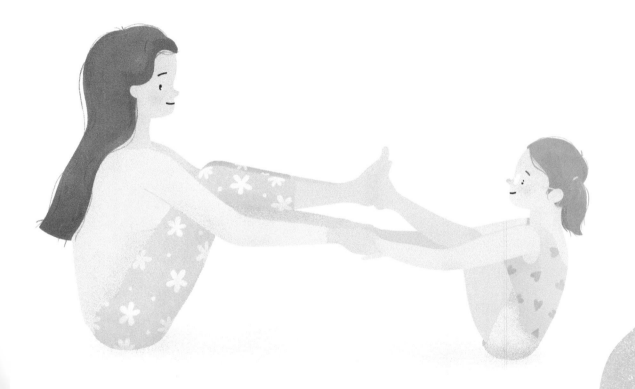

DOUBLE PLANK

7 AND UP

 ENERGIZING

 STRENGTHENING

This is a challenging pose that integrates strength and teamwork at once. In most cases, Double Plank will rely on the grown-up being Partner A on the ground in Plank to initiate the pose. Partner A must be able to hold Partner B up in the pose, which requires trust. For those who enjoy a physical and mental challenge, set a timer for a specific amount of time and hold steady until the allotted time is up. Remember to focus on the breath!

1. Partner A starts in Plank (page 54).

2. Partner B stands over Partner A, facing the opposite direction and with one leg on each side of Partner A's calves.

3. Partner B folds down to grab the backs of Partner A's heels and ankles.

4. Partner B steps both feet back and gently places her feet on Partner A's upper back or shoulders.

5. Both partners take a few deep breaths here and feel strong and powerful in this partner pose.

6. To release, Partner B steps her feet down on either side of Partner A and slowly lifts her hands off Partner A's heels, rising back to standing. Partner A lowers to the ground.

TIP

- Double Plank can be taken to the next level with a Double Plank push-up. When both partners feel steady and strong in Double Plank, Partner A can practice a Yoga Push-Up (page 56) with the added challenge of Partner B holding Plank pose above her. Try one double push-up to begin, and if you're feeling strong, add in more.

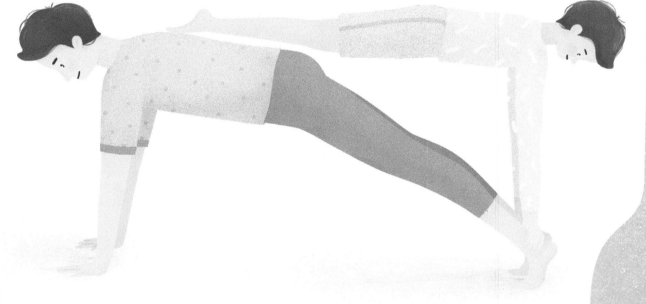

CHAPTER

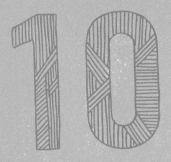

10

YOGA
GAMES

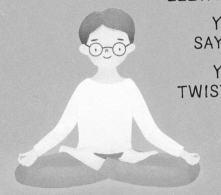

Games are a great way to engage kids with yoga poses, breathing activities, and even meditations. These games are perfect to practice at home with two or three kids or a larger group. Starting off your yoga session with a game will get everyone's attention and ease kids into the yoga frame of mind. If you find a game your kids love, be sure to use it repeatedly in your yoga practice, so they can remember to look forward to it. You can also entice kids to a session by promising one of their favorite games. These games are simple and can be done at home or on the go, for any amount of time.

FOLLOW ME

ALL AGES

 REJUVENATING

This game is a fun way to begin a yoga session. It engages kids with simple, rhythmic moves and helps them get focused. Ask kids to follow you and lead them through a series of stomps, claps, snaps, silly dance moves—you name it! Kids love the rhythm and imitation of this game, and you don't have to use your voice. Follow Me can seamlessly lead into your first yoga pose of the session.

1. Start in Mountain (page 40) and take a deep breath.

2. Stomp your right foot twice. Repeat this action a couple of times as kids follow along.

3. Repeat on the left side.

4. Clap your hands twice.

5. Clap your hands twice, then stomp the right foot, followed by the left foot.

6. Demonstrate a deep breath: inhale and reach the arms overhead with a clap at the top, exhale, and draw the palms down together at the sternum.

7. Make a silly movement, like wiggling your entire body.

8. Keep going with any movements or noises, and end Follow Me with a yoga pose.

ELEVATORS

ALL AGES

 REJUVENATING

This game is fast-paced and fun and helps strengthen the core muscles and lower body. It's a play on Chair pose (page 72), but kids might not even notice the challenge! Kids love this one because it requires focus and involves a sense of anticipation. Everyone pretends they are an elevator as you call out different floors. The lower the elevator gets, the deeper kids go into their Chair pose, getting closer and closer to the ground.

1. Stand in the middle of your yoga mat and face your yoga partner or teammates.

2. Announce a floor between 1 and 10.

3. The lower the floor, the closer everyone needs to get to the ground, crouching down deeper and deeper into Chair pose (page 72).

4. Have some fun moving quickly between floors on distant levels, like 1 to 10! Be silly and add a high floor, like 5 to 33, jumping high into the air as you announce it.

5. Suddenly hold a floor and have everybody freeze.

6. After a few rounds, ask the other person to be the leader. In a bigger group, trade off until everyone has had a chance to lead.

YOGI SAYS

ALL AGES

 REJUVENATING

This is the yoga version of Simon Says. Create any variation of the instructions below using your basic yoga poses (see chapter 4, page 39). Here is simply a sample script. The game will come alive with your personal creativity. Before you start, observe the energy level of the room to decide if you want a fast, high-energy session or a calming combination of poses. When it's time to end the game, use slow, deep breaths to slow the game down.

1. Yogi says "Down Dog."
2. Yogi says "Lift your right leg."
3. Yogi says "Place your right leg back on the floor."
4. "Lift your left leg." (See if anybody gets tricked.)
5. Yogi says "Candle."
6. Yogi says "Light your candle."
7. Yogi says "Blow out your candle."
8. Yogi says "Tree"
9. Yogi says "Criss-Cross"
10. Yogi says "Take two long, deep breaths."
11. After a few rounds, let someone else be the leader.

YOGI TWISTER

ALL AGES

 REJUVENATING

This is an easy way to engage kids and trick them into warming up the body or doing yoga poses. This game relies on one simple instruction: the body parts you call out are the only ones allowed on the yoga mat. Kids love the anticipation of what comes next in this game. They make great leaders of Yogi Twister as well. Here's an example script.

1. Just your belly.
2. One hand, one foot.
3. Two hands, two feet.
4. Two elbows, two knees.
5. Just your bottom.
6. Two feet.
7. One foot.
8. After several rounds, let someone else be the leader.

STRIKE A POSE

ALL AGES

 REJUVENATING

Freeze dance for yogis! This is a great way to help kids memorize the names of different poses or try new poses in a fun, energetic setting.

1. Crank up some fun music. Make sure it's something both you and your child enjoy.

2. Dance around and have fun.

3. Press "pause," and when the music stops, move into any yoga pose. Call out a few yoga pose suggestions if it seems like your child is stuck.

4. Crank up the music again and repeat.

MIRROR GAME

ALL AGES

 CALMING

This game promotes focus, cooperation, and mindful observation. It's also a silent game, which makes it a great choice for setting the tone for relaxation or meditation.

1. Have partners face each other on a yoga mat and make it clear that this is a silent game, so no talking is allowed.

2. One partner begins with a simple movement as the other partner mirrors the movement.

3. Continue using slow, mindful movements and breath, eventually including some yoga poses.

4. Set a timer and switch leaders when the time's up.

5. To integrate relaxation into the game, you can end in meditation or Rest pose (page 182).

YOGA STORYTIME 1

ALL AGES

 REJUVENATING

This game is great for integrating storytelling and imagination into a yoga session. Below is a sample story and sequence. Feel free to use this one or create your own stories with special places and objects meaningful to you and your child.

1. Explain that you are going to tell a yoga story, and every time you mention a yoga pose, it's a signal for everyone to get into the pose and hold it for five seconds.

2. Once upon a time, I set out on an epic adventure. I wanted to see the temples in Japan. I bought my ticket and boarded a large **Boat** (page 94).

3. We sailed for several days before we came upon a storm. The boat **rocked and shook** (rock and shake your Boat), but thankfully we made it through.

TIPS

- Lower the forearms to the ground to become a Dolphin. Dolphin strengthens the arms and holds the same form in the legs, hips, and spine as Down Dog.
- Turn the hands out to the side to become a Seal. Add in seal barks with little ones to gain additional time opening the upper body and chest.

4. The sun shone through the clouds and all was well. We even saw a pod of **Dolphins** (see tip). But just as we all began to clap and cheer, some pirates boarded the **Boat** and told us we would have to walk the **Plank** (page 54).

5. We were scared, but the pirates were persistent: they made us all leave the **Boat** and walk the **Plank** anyway!

6. Some of the passengers were struggling to swim, but then we floated past a **Bridge** (page 60). Some of the swimmers climbed up to safety. I noticed some **Seals** (see tip) sunning themselves on the rocks by the **Bridge**. I told them what happened and, to my surprise, they sprang into action!

7. They told all the passengers to climb on their backs and they would swim all the way back to the **Boat**. When we arrived, the pirates were having a wild party, even using the **Plank** as a diving board!

8. The **Seals** jumped onto the deck and barked so fiercely at the pirates that they got scared! The pirates jumped off the **Boat** and swam back to their own ship. We all had a delicious dinner in celebration. Once we pulled into the harbor in Nagoya, Japan, we hugged and thanked the **Seals** once more as they jumped off the **Boat** and swam off, joining the **Dolphins** in the distance.

9. Later that night, it was time for everyone to close their eyes, take a few deep breaths, and **Rest** (page 182).

YOGA STORYTIME 2

ALL AGES

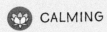 CALMING

This is a creative way to weave yoga into reading time. Here's a tip: You can use almost any book to create a yoga adventure. The example here demonstrates how to do this with an Eric Carle book. As you tell the story, let your creativity and love of reading guide you. For older kids ages 11 to 12, you can ask them to choose a yoga sequence at the end of each chapter of a book they're reading. This gives them more choice and freedom and gets them moving during downtime.

1. For the best results, choose a book with repetition of a phrase, name, or word like *Brown Bear, Goodnight Moon,* or *Ada Twist.*

2. Choose an activity or series of activities to integrate as you read the book. If you're reading at night and hope to create a calming effect, choose meditations or breathing exercises. In the morning, try some twisting poses to get everyone stretching.

3. We'll use *Brown Bear* by Eric Carle as an example.

4. Say something like the following: "We're going to read *Brown Bear* today and every time we hear the phrase 'What do you see?' we're going to take a big Bubble Breath (page 36) in and out. Are you ready?"

TIP

- If your child knows how to read, ask him to read the book and lead you through a storytime yoga practice.

5. Begin reading the story and when you get to "What do you see?" pause and take a nice, deep Bubble Breath.

6. If you'd like to create a more energizing effect, integrate more active poses like Down Dog (page 52), Tree (page 134), or even a yoga sequence.

CHAPTER

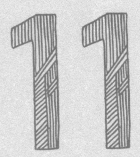

11

RELAXATION

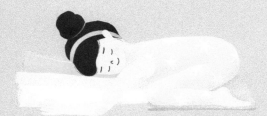

Relaxation is an essential component to yoga practice. When we learn to practice relaxation as an integrated part of yoga, it sends the message that self-care and relaxation are just as important as performance and activity. With an integrated relaxation practice, you can guide your family to value relaxation just as much as the games, sequences, and more active poses. Be sure to include relaxation in all your yoga sessions for a truly nourishing experience.

REST POSE

ALL AGES

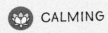 CALMING

The final yoga pose in most sequences, Rest pose restores and relaxes the body. Rest is often sought after by kids in yoga. Once you teach the pose, you might find them asking about it often when practicing yoga: "When do we get to take a nap?" If your child asks this question, don't hesitate to oblige—she may need more opportunities to relax and unwind. And there's nothing wrong with taking a moment in stillness.

1. Start by lying on your back on the yoga mat.

2. Put your hands by your sides and create space in the body by separating your ankles by at least 12 inches, if not more. Let your feet relax and fall to the sides.

3. Gently arch your back and draw your shoulder blades under your body.

4. Relax everything into the ground, especially the back of your head, and all your limbs. Feel your body go heavy.

5. Close your eyes as you continue to relax the body.

6. Let go of everything. No need to focus on the breath or the body; simply allow the body and mind to rest and be still.

TIP

- Rest pose is not always easy, even though it only requires lying on the ground and breathing. When your mind races, Rest might feel like one of the most challenging poses yet. The first step to relaxing when you have a racing mind is to accept the fact that you have a racing mind and tell yourself it's okay! Then use a method that helps you slow down your thoughts, such as Balloon Breath (page 29) or Counting Meditation (page 246).

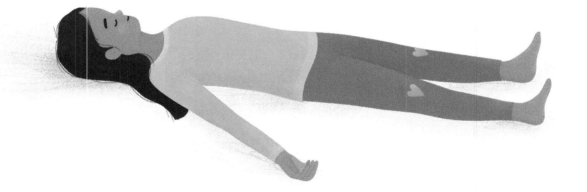

BODY SCAN: SHORT VERSION

5 AND UP

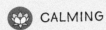 CALMING

Bringing awareness to specific areas of the body can help soothe and relax the body. In this relaxation exercise, you'll close your eyes and bring kind attention to yourself as you scan the body. Notice how you feel in each finger, toe, joint, and muscle. If you find an area that is tense, focus on relaxing it. If you notice yourself becoming critical of an ache or pain or a certain part of the body, simply say to yourself "thanks, but no thanks," and send some love to that body part as you tell your inner critic to take a hike! Read these instructions aloud to your child or record yourself (or your child) and use the audio version to practice the body scan together. Make sure you are nice and warm when practicing this pose. You can have blankets on hand to cover up.

1. Start by lying down on your back on the yoga mat. If your lower back feels at all uncomfortable, place a rolled blanket or towel underneath your knees to elevate them.

2. Take a deep inhale and exhale and imagine your body sinking deeper into the ground.

3. As you take slow, gentle breaths, bring your attention to the back of your head. Imagine adding five pounds to the weight of your head to make it even heavier against the floor.

4. Bring your attention to your belly. If it's tense, release the muscles.

5. Notice your jaw. If it's clenched, separate the top and bottom teeth slightly as you relax your jaw muscles.

6. Allow your neck and shoulders to relax.

7. Breathe gently and notice your right arm, then the right hand, and then the fingers.

8. Notice your left arm, hand, and fingers.

9. Bring your attention to your right leg, then the right foot, and even the toes.

10. Notice the left leg, foot, and toes.

11. Shift your attention from any single body part to the entire body, breathing and relaxed on the ground.

12. Take a few deep breaths and wiggle your fingers and toes to activate the body.

13. Gently draw your knees into your chest and roll to one side.

14. Slowly press your hands into the ground to lift up to a seated position.

BODY SCAN: LONG VERSION

7 AND UP

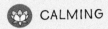 CALMING

When you have more time to dedicate to a body scan, unwind and nourish the body with this meditative scan. This practice is deeply soothing and meditative. As you consciously relax specific parts of the body for extended periods, you are training those areas of the body to release tension. This practice reduces stress and calms the nervous system. Read these instructions aloud to your child or record yourself (or your child) and use an audio version to practice the body scan together. Make sure you are nice and warm when practicing this pose. You can have blankets on hand to cover up.

1. Start by lying down on your back on the yoga mat. If your lower back feels at all uncomfortable, place a rolled blanket or towel underneath your knees to elevate them.

2. Take a deep inhale and exhale and imagine your body sinking deeper into the ground.

3. As you take slow, gentle breaths, bring your attention to the back of your head. Imagine adding five pounds to the weight of your head to make it even heavier against the floor.

4. Bring your attention to your belly. If it's tense, release the muscles.

5. Draw your attention to the space between your eyebrows, relaxing the tiny muscles there.

6. Soften the inner corners of the eyes.

7. Notice the roof of the mouth.

8. Bring your attention to your nostrils and feel the air enter and exit as you breathe gently.

9. Bring your attention to the belly. If it's tense, release the muscles.

10. Notice your jaw and separate the top and bottom teeth slightly as you relax the muscles around the jaw.

11. Allow your neck and shoulders to relax.

12. Breathe gently and notice the right shoulder, elbow, and wrist.

13. Feel the right fingers. Begin with the thumb and spend a moment of awareness on each finger all the way to the pinky.

14. Breathe gently and notice the left shoulder, elbow, and wrist.

15. Feel the left fingers. Begin with the thumb and spend a moment of awareness on each finger all the way to the pinky.

16. Bring your attention to the right hip.

17. Breathe gently as you notice the right thigh, knee, and ankle joint.

18. Notice the right foot and spend a moment of awareness on each toe.

19. Bring your attention to the left hip.

20. Breathe gently as you notice the left thigh, knee, and ankle joint.

21. Notice the left foot and spend a moment of awareness on each toe.

22. Shift your attention from any single body part to the entire body, breathing and relaxed on the ground.

23. Take a few deep breaths and wiggle your fingers and toes to activate the body.

24. Gently draw your knees into your chest and roll to one side.

25. Slowly press your hands into the ground to lift up to a seated position.

TENSE AND RELEASE

ALL AGES

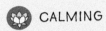 CALMING

There are calming and therapeutic benefits to exaggerating the tension in the body. This practice is more formally known as "progressive muscle relaxation." When we exaggerate tension, we acknowledge the body's tension and immediately allow it to release. This can be especially helpful if you feel excited, angry, anxious, or restless. Make sure to use a sense of humor here as you squeeze and scrunch the muscles in the body.

1. Start by lying down on your back on the yoga mat. If your lower back feels at all uncomfortable, place a rolled blanket or towel underneath your knees to elevate them.

2. Take a deep inhale and exhale and imagine your body sinking deeper into the ground.

3. Inhale and squeeze the muscles in your belly as tight as possible. Keep squeezing for a few seconds. Exhale and release and relax.

4. Squeeze the right hand, making a fist. Squeeze tightly and keep squeezing up the forearm, bicep, and all the way up to the right shoulder. Release the hold, relaxing the shoulder and arm.

5. Squeeze the left hand, making a fist. Squeeze tightly and keep squeezing up the forearm, bicep, and all the way up to the left shoulder. Release the hold, relaxing the shoulder and arm.

6. Scrunch up the entire face, tensing the face muscles and the jaw. Have fun with this. It can look very silly. Release and relax.

7. Squeeze all the muscles down your right leg. Then the right foot and even the toes. Squeeze tightly, then release.

8. Squeeze all the muscles down your left leg. Then the right foot and even the toes. Squeeze tightly, then release.

9. Inhale, and with all your strength, squeeze all the muscles in your body, tensing the entire body as much as possible. Exhale and release.

10. Take a few slow, deep breaths.

11. Gently draw your knees into your chest and roll to one side.

12. Slowly press your hands into the ground to lift up to a seated position.

LEGS UP THE WALL

ALL AGES

 CALMING

 REJUVENATING

This is a restorative yoga pose that can be practiced for as long as it feels good for you—from a few minutes to half an hour or more. This pose is believed to help with anxiety and stress, so it's a great relaxation to practice the night before a big test or game. It's also a wonderful way to wind down your yoga session. You may want to add extra lift under your lower back with some folded blankets.

1. Place your yoga mat with one short end against a wall.

2. Have a folded blanket or two on hand to provide extra lift under the lower back.

3. Sit sideways against the wall with the left hip pointed toward the wall.

4. Draw your knees in, and using your hands on the ground by your sides, turn and lift the legs straight up the wall so that your feet reach up to the sky.

5. Release your back onto the mat and use your arms to scoot your bottom closer to the wall, so your body forms an "L" shape against the wall.

6. With the back released entirely on the mat, drop your hands by your sides or onto your belly.

7. Breathe gently and allow the entire body to release and relax. Feel gravity pulling you down and your legs growing lighter.

8. Stay here for a few minutes or longer, breathing gently and allowing gravity to assist the body in deep relaxation.

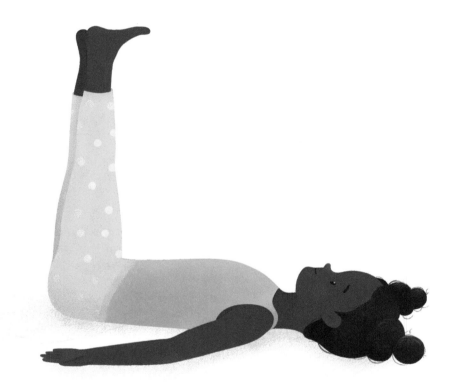

WAVES VISUALIZATION

5 AND UP

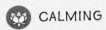 CALMING

This is a soothing relaxation practice that can be deeply personal and effective. The visualization helps us identify our feelings and connects us to the rhythm of our breath to wash away any stress, fears, or anxiety. Kids tend to love the beach, which means they love this summery visualization any time of year.

1. Start by lying on your back on the mat.

2. Imagine you are standing on the sand near the ocean. The sand feels wonderful beneath your feet, so warm and soft. It's a perfect day with just the right amount of sunshine. Feel the warm sun on your skin, and see the sunlight sparkling on the water.

3. As you stand here, notice a beautiful rhythm to the waves as they glide onto shore and ease back into the ocean.

4. Start to match your breathing to the rhythm of the waves. Breathe in (pause)—and out.

TIP

- If you and your child have visited the ocean together, you can recall the sights and sounds you saw to help set a calming mood. You can also create variations of this practice, imagining different types of weather or details about the beach or waves. At the end of the visualization, you can ask your child to share what qualities he chose to breathe in and out. But never force your child to share, demonstrating respect for privacy.

5. As you're breathing, breathe in something that feels good and you might want more of inside you, like joy or gratitude or love.

6. Breathe out anything negative like fear or insecurity and let it go.

7. Keep breathing in and saying just that one thing that feels nurturing. For example, breathe in calm, breathe out sad.

SUPPORTED CHILD'S POSE

ALL AGES

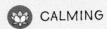 CALMING

This pose builds on the calming nature of Child's Pose (page 46) for a soothing resting position. It is extremely comforting to have the weight of the body supported with the belly to the ground. The softness of the bolster or pillow allows the body to completely relax and the mind to let go. This is a great pose to suggest when a child is worked up or overwhelmed.

1. Start on your knees with the knees hip-width apart on the floor and toes touching behind you.

2. Widen your knees and place the bolster or a pillow in front of you lengthwise on the mat between your knees.

3. Allow the torso and chest to relax down onto the bolster or pillow. Adjust as necessary, adding more pillows for additional height and comfort.

4. Turn your head to one side and breathe gently for any length of time, from 30 seconds to three minutes (set a timer).

5. Repeat with your head turned to the opposite side.

6. To release, gently press the hands down onto the floor and lift up to a seated position.

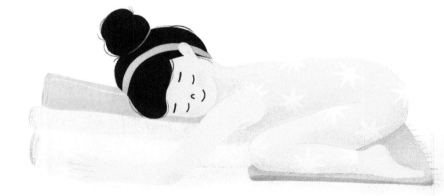

YIN BUTTERFLY

7 AND UP

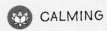 CALMING

Yin yoga is a practice of stillness and awareness. There are no goals to deepen the pose or push further. Instead, holding poses in stillness leads to a natural softening in the muscles and in the mind. Pay attention to your breathing in this pose. When you notice your mind wandering, simply name whatever is happening: planning, remembering, imagining, and so on. Then bring your attention back to your breathing.

1. Sit on a folded blanket, bolster, or pillow.

2. Shift your weight forward, bend your knees, press the soles of your feet together, and get into Butterfly (page 86).

3. Place your heels approximately 12 inches away from your hips. With your hands on your ankles, bend forward from the hips with a long spine and lean forward as far as is comfortable, then relax your head and neck and curl down toward your heels. If your hips and hamstrings are tight, you may be quite elevated in this position, and that is great.

4. Rest your head in the arches of the feet. If you can't reach, stack your fists to support your head, or cup your head in the hands while your elbows rest on your feet.

5. Breathe gently for three to five minutes.

6. Inhale as you come up, then stretch your legs forward and lean back on your hands. Exhale and relax. Feel still for a few breaths here.

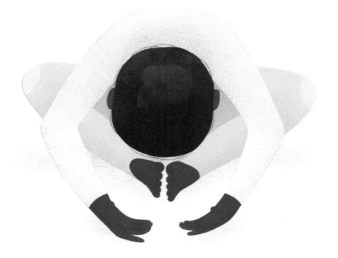

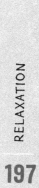

CHAPTER

12

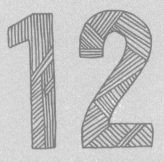

YOGA SEQUENCES

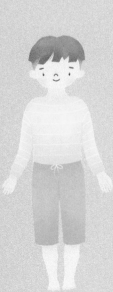

Yoga sequences are designed as groups of poses linked together by the breath. Sequences vary in length, and the yoga poses are chosen to sequentially move the body toward deep relaxation in Rest pose (page 182). Notice your personal preferences as you practice yoga sequences and be aware of how and why your preferences might change. For example, you may enjoy a more active sequence early in the morning and a more calming and still practice in the afternoon or evening. For others, the exact opposite might be true, as a more physically active practice may help them unwind after a long day. There is no right or wrong sequence to practice. It's all about listening to your body and mind. You can assist your child in this reflection by asking how she feels after a sequence or offering to try something different if you notice something just isn't working for her. Be flexible and adapt your routines as you go.

SUN SALUTE 1

ALL AGES

 REJUVENATING

Sun Salutes are the building blocks of a yoga sequence. Enjoy the rhythm of the inhales and exhales as you move through the cycle of poses. These are wonderful sequences to do first thing in the morning to greet the sun. As you move, focus on the breath and the body and try to quiet the mind. The idea is to let go and flow.

1. Start in a seated position for one to three minutes, breathing gently. Allow the eyes to close or take the gaze down, but keep the neck and spine long.

2. Inhale and make your way into **Table Top** (page 44).

3. Exhale into **Down Dog** (page 52).

4. Inhale, **Plank** (page 54).

5. Exhale, step to the front of the mat, **Forward Fold** (page 42).

6. Inhale, lift the torso halfway up, and exhale, release back down into the fold.

7. Inhale, reach the arms up and rise into **Mountain** (page 40).

8. Exhale, **Forward Fold**.

9. Inhale, lift the torso halfway up. Exhale, release back down into **Forward Fold**.

10. Inhale, step back into **Plank**.

11. Exhale, lower the knees, thighs, belly, and chest to the ground, placing your hands by the sides of the ribs.

12. Inhale, lift into **Cobra** (page 58).

13. Press the hands and feet down firmly into the ground, engage the core muscles, and exhale, lift into **Down Dog**.

14. Inhale, step into **Forward Fold**.

15. Reach the arms overhead and exhale, release the hands by your side in **Mountain**.

16. Repeat as many times as you'd like.

SUN SALUTE 2

ALL AGES

 REJUVENATING

A foundational sequence in yoga practice, Sun Salute 2 opens the hips and upper body and creates a rhythmic pattern with the breath.

1. Start in **Mountain** (page 40).
2. Bend the knees into **Chair** (page 72) and take a few rounds of breath.
3. Exhale, **Forward Fold** (page 42).
4. Inhale, lift the torso halfway up, exhale, **Forward Fold**.
5. Inhale, **Plank** (page 54).
6. Exhale, lower the knees to the ground.
7. Inhale, lift the knees, thighs, and upper body as you press the hands down by your sides, **Up Dog** (page 120).
8. Exhale, press the hands down, engage the core, and lift the hips into **Down Dog** (page 52).
9. Inhale, step the right leg forward toward the top of the mat, **Warrior 1** (page 66).
10. Exhale, step back into **Plank**.
11. Inhale, **Up Dog**.
12. Exhale, **Down Dog**.
13. Inhale, step the left foot forward toward the top of the mat, **Warrior 1**.

14. Exhale, step back into **Plank**.

15. Inhale, **Up Dog**.

16. Exhale, press the hands down, engage the core, and lift the hips back into **Down Dog**.

17. Inhale, step to the front of your mat, and exhale, **Forward Fold**.

18. Inhale, lift and extend the torso halfway up, exhale, **Forward Fold**.

19. Inhale, lift the arms and elongate the spine, and maintain a bend in the knees as you lift into **Chair**.

20. Exhale, **Mountain**.

21. Repeat two to four more times.

SIMPLE SEQUENCE 1

ALL AGES

 REJUVENATING

This is a well-rounded practice that includes a nice warm-up Down Dog (page 52) and Plank (page 54). The sequence then moves into standing poses like Star (page 64) and Triangle (page 70) followed by twists and seated poses. This versatile sequence is great for morning or after school with rejuvenating effects.

1. Start in **Criss-Cross** (page 100), inhaling and exhaling a few times to connect to your breath.

2. On an exhale, take **Child's Pose** (page 46), then inhale to **Table Top** (page 44), and repeat this three times.

3. Inhale to **Table Top**, exhale to **Down Dog** (page 52), and repeat this three times.

4. Inhale in **Down Dog** and exhale to **Plank** (page 54), and repeat this three times.

5. Inhale in **Down Dog** and exhale, step the right foot forward to the front of the mat, lower the left knee, and take a round of breath in **Low Lunge** (page 76).

6. On an exhale, take **Down Dog**.

7. Inhale in **Down Dog** and exhale, step the left foot forward to the front of the mat, lower the right knee, and take a round of breath in **Low Lunge**, opposite side.

8. On an exhale, take **Down Dog**.

9. Inhale, step to the middle of your mat, **Mountain** (page 40).

10. Turn to face the side of the mat and step the feet apart about three feet into **Star** (page 64).

11. Turn the left foot in to an approximate 45-degree angle and reach the arms wide. Exhale into **Triangle** (page 70). Take a few rounds of breath in **Triangle**, and on an exhale, engage the core and lift back into **Star**.

12. Now turn the right foot in to an approximate 45-degree angle and reach the arms wide. Exhale into **Triangle**, opposite side. Take a few rounds of breath in **Triangle**, and on an exhale, engage the core and lift back into **Star**.

13. Take **Criss-Cross** and reach the arms high into the air on an inhale, and on the exhale, turn the torso toward the right, reaching the right arm back and fingertips to the floor, into **Seated Twist** (page 114) on the right side.

14. On an exhale, take **Criss-Cross**. Inhale to reach the arms high into the air, and on the exhale, turn the torso toward the left, reaching the left arm back and fingertips to the floor, into **Seated Twist**, left side.

15. Roll onto your back with your knees up and feet pressing into the ground. Gently tuck the shoulder blades underneath you. Lift the hips up, and on an inhale, take **Bridge** (page 60). Exhale and lower the hips down.

16. Lift up to a seated position, bend the knees out to the side, and press the soles of the feet together for **Butterfly** (page 86). Take a few rounds of breath here.

17. Extend the right leg, gently press the left foot against the right inner thigh into **Dragonfly** (page 90), and stay for a few rounds of breath.

18. Switch sides and extend your left leg out, gently pressing the right foot against the inner left thigh into **Dragonfly**, opposite side. Stay for a few rounds of breath.

19. Slowly release and take a comfortable position lying down.

20. **Waves Visualization** (page 192).

SIMPLE SEQUENCE 2

ALL AGES

 REJUVENATING

This sequence stretches the quadricep and calf muscles with Low Lunges (page 76) and opens the groin muscles with Triangle (page 70) and Wide-Legged Forward Fold (page 110). The Warrior poses build focus and strength to relieve stress, and the practice ultimately unwinds in Rest pose (page 182).

1. Sit in **Criss-Cross** (page 100) and practice your preferred meditation (see chapter 13, page 233) for two minutes, setting a timer.

2. When the timer goes off, make your way into **Table Top** (page 44).

3. Inhale, **Cow** (page 50), exhale **Cat** (page 48). Repeat three times.

4. From **Table Top**, step the right foot forward into **Low Lunge** (page 76) for a few breaths.

5. Inhale, reach your arms overhead, exhale, and twist to the right, reaching the left hand to the right knee, **Low Lunge Twist** (page 116). Stay for a few breaths.

6. On an exhale, step back to **Plank** (page 54).

7. Inhale, slowly lower the body to the ground. Press the hands and feet down, and lift up to **Cobra** (page 58).

8. Exhale, lift the hips up and back to **Down Dog** (page 52).

9. Inhale, step the right foot forward, **Warrior 1** (page 66).

10. Exhale, reach the arms out to the side, **Warrior 2** (page 68). Hold for a few rounds of breath.

11. Inhale, turn the heel to lift to the ceiling, ball of the foot pressing down into the ground, set the hands down to the mat, and exhale. Lower the left knee to the ground, **Low Lunge**, hold.

12. Inhale, reach the arms up, exhale, twist the torso to the right and press the left hand to the right knee, **Low Lunge Twist**. Take a few rounds of breath.

13. On an exhale, step back into **Plank**.

14. Set the knees and chest down on the ground.

15. Inhale, press the hands and tops of the feet into the ground, and lift into **Cobra** (page 58).

16. Exhale, lift the hips, and press back into **Down Dog**. Hold for a couple of breaths.

17. On an exhale, step your left foot forward and angle your right foot to 45 degrees as you lift into **Warrior 1**.

18. Exhale, extend the arms to the side, **Warrior 2**.

19. Inhale, turn the heel to lift to the ceiling, ball of the foot pressing down into the ground, set the hands down to the mat, and exhale. Lower the right knee to the ground, **Low Lunge**. Hold for a moment.

20. Inhale, reach the arms up, exhale, twist the torso to the left and press the right hand to the left knee, **Low Lunge Twist**. Take a few rounds of breath here.

21. On an exhale, step back into **Plank**. Inhale.

22. Exhale, **Down Dog**.

23. Inhale, step the feet forward into **Mountain** (page 40) for a few rounds of breath.

24. Inhale, step the right leg back, reach the left arm forward, and lean forward into **Triangle** (page 70) for a round of breath.

25. Keeping the legs wide and straight, stay low and move the torso to the right until your body is facing the side of the yoga mat. Turn both feet to face forward and release the head and neck into **Wide-Legged Forward Fold** (page 110). On an exhale, gently lift the torso up, standing upright with the legs wide on the mat.

26. Inhale, angle the left foot behind you to 45 degrees, reach the right arm forward, and lean forward into **Triangle** for a round of breath.

continued

27. Extend the right leg, and gently press the left foot against the right inner thigh, sinking down into **Dragonfly** (page 90). Stay for a few rounds of breath.

28. Switch sides, extending the left leg now and gently pressing the right foot against the left inner thigh, sinking into **Dragonfly**, opposite side. Stay for a few rounds of breath.

29. Release the entire body to the yoga mat, lying on your back.

30. Rest the hands by the sides and move the legs apart, separating the ankles by at least 12 inches, and settle into **Rest Pose** (page 182).

31. Relax everything into the ground, especially the back of the head, and all the limbs.

32. Close your eyes as you release.

33. Let go of everything. No need to focus on the breath or body anymore; simply allow the body and mind to rest and be.

INTERMEDIATE SEQUENCE 1

5 AND UP

 REJUVENATING

This refreshing sequence provides a fun moment of connection with Double Tree (page 156) and ends with a nourishing Body Scan: Short Version (page 184). It's the perfect way to start or end the day!

1. **Concentration Meditation** (page 234).

2. Stand at the front of your mat in **Mountain** (page 40).

3. Step the left foot toward the back of the mat and set the left knee on the ground for **Low Lunge** (page 76). Clasp the hands behind the back, drawing the shoulder blades down the back to open the front chest.

4. Release the hands, lift the left knee.

5. Press the hands down into the mat and send the right foot back to meet the left as you lift the hips into **Down Dog** (page 52). Take a couple rounds of breath.

6. Step the right foot forward toward the front of the mat, bend the right knee, angle the left foot at a 45-degree angle into **Warrior 2** (page 68).

7. Keep the legs in the same position, take the right forearm to the right thigh, and extend the left arm overhead into **Side Angle** (page 78).

continued

8. Straighten the right leg and angle the hips back to the left as you lean the torso to the right into **Triangle** (page 70) for a round of breath.

9. Lift back into **Warrior 2** (page 68), circle the hands down to the mat and step both feet back for **Plank** (page 54).

10. Inhale, lower the body to the ground, and press the hands and feet down, lifting the torso into **Cobra**.

11. Exhale, lift the hips up and back to **Down Dog** (page 52).

12. Step the feet forward to **Mountain** at the front of your mat.

13. Step the right foot toward the back of the mat and set the right knee on the ground for **Low Lunge** (page 76). Clasp the hands behind the back, drawing the shoulder blades down the back to open the front chest. Release the hands, lift the knee.

14. Press the hands down into the mat and send the left foot back to meet the right as you lift the hips into **Down Dog**. Take a couple of rounds of breath.

15. Step the left foot forward toward the top of the mat, bend the left knee, angle the right foot at a 45-degree angle into **Warrior 2**.

16. Keep the legs in the same position, take the left forearm to the left thigh, and extend the right arm overhead into **Side Angle**.

17. Straighten the left leg and angle the hips back to the right as you lean the torso to the left into **Triangle** for a round of breath.

18. Lift back into **Warrior 2**, circle the hands down to the mat and step both feet back for **Plank**.

19. Inhale, lower the body to the ground, and press the hands and feet down, lifting the torso into **Cobra**.

20. Exhale, lift the hips up and back to **Down Dog**.

21. Step the feet forward to **Mountain** at the front of your mat.

22. Find a partner and face each other, balancing in **Tree** (page 134) for **Double Tree** (page 156; remember to mirror each other and hold hands at the top of the pose).

23. Take a few deep breaths, release your hands, and set the elevated foot down.

24. Repeat **Double Tree** on the other side.

25. Return to standing at the front of your mat, **Mountain**.

26. Reach the arms up and over-head, extend the torso forward into **Forward Fold** (page 42), hold for a few rounds of breath.

27. Place your hands on the mat and lower the knees, scooting them into **Table Top** (page 44).

28. Press the hands down and send the hips back toward the feet, **Child's Pose** (page 46).

29. Roll onto your back with your knees up and feet pressing into the ground. Gently tuck the shoulder blades underneath you. Exhale, lift the hips into **Bridge** (page 60). Exhale and lower the hips down.

30. Hug your knees into your chest and grab the top of each foot with the corresponding hand for **Happy Baby** (page 92).

31. Release the feet, extend the legs, and relax the entire body.

32. End with **Body Scan: Short Version** (page 184).

INTERMEDIATE SEQUENCE 2

5 AND UP

 REJUVENATING

 STRENGTHENING

This sequence begins with a meditation to ground and focus your practice. Active standing poses and core work in Boat (page 94), with a focus on the breath, lead to the fun balancing pose Dancer (page 138). Hero pose (page 96) and the Waves Visualization (page 192) counterbalance the strength-building aspect of the sequence and round out the practice with relaxation.

1. Sit on the mat in simple **Criss-Cross** (page 100).

2. Silent **Concentration Meditation** (page 234) for three minutes.

3. Step the left foot back, lower the left knee to the ground, **Low Lunge** (page 76).

4. Clasp the hands behind the back, drawing the shoulder blades down the back to open the front chest.

5. Release the hands, lift the left knee.

6. Press the hands down to the mat, send the right foot back to meet the left, lift the hips into **Down Dog** (page 52).

7. Step the right foot forward toward the front of the mat, bend the right knee, and angle the left foot at a 45-degree angle into **Warrior 2** (page 68).

8. Keep the legs in the same position, take the right forearm to the right thigh, and extend the left arm overhead into **Side Angle** (page 78).

9. Straighten the right leg and angle the hips back to the left as you lean the torso to the right into **Triangle** (page 70) for a round of breath.

10. Lift back into **Warrior 2**, circle the hands down to the mat, and step both feet back for **Plank** (page 54).

11. Inhale, lower the body to the ground, press the hands and feet down, and lift the torso into **Cobra** (page 58).

12. Press the hands and feet down, lift the hips up into **Down Dog**.

13. Walk the feet forward to the top of the mat, **Mountain** (page 40).

14. Step the right foot toward the back of the mat and set the right knee on the ground for **Low Lunge**. Clasp the hands behind the back, drawing the shoulder blades down the back to open the front chest. Release the hands, lift the knee.

15. Press the hands down to the mat, send the right foot back to meet the left, and lift the hips into **Down Dog**. Take a couple of rounds of breath here.

16. Step the left foot forward toward the front of the mat, bend the left knee, and angle the right foot at a 45-degree angle into **Warrior 2**.

17. Keep the legs in the same position, take the left forearm to the left thigh, and extend the right arm overhead into **Side Angle**.

18. Straighten the left leg and angle the hips back to the right as you lean the torso to the left into **Triangle** for a round of breath.

19. Lift back into **Warrior 2**, circle the hands down to the mat, and step both feet back for **Plank**.

20. Lower the knees and sit back on your heels. Find a partner and face each other, connecting with each other's feet for **Double Boat** (page 164).

21. Continue to press the soles of the feet against one another, creating leverage as you hold hands to build a deeper connection in the pose.

22. Lift and lengthen through the back. If straight knees are not possible, simply stay in the pose with the knees bent.

23. Take a few deep breaths and release the hands and the feet to the ground.

24. Step to the front of your mat for **Mountain**.

continued

25. If you have more time, add in **Sun Salute 1** (page 200).

26. Breathe in and shift your weight onto the right foot, lifting your left heel up and back toward your bottom. Exhale and reach the left arm back to grab the outside of the left foot, **Dancer** (page 138).

27. Lower the left foot and step your feet wide enough apart that you can squat your bottom down toward the ground. Be liberal with the amount of space you give yourself.

28. Take an inhale, and as you exhale, squat down toward the ground into **Frog** (page 82).

29. Press your palms together at your sternum and take a few deep breaths in **Frog**.

30. Sit back on your heels with your knees forward for **Hero** (page 96). Place a rolled blanket or towel between your calves and thighs if you need additional support.

31. Breathe in and elongate the spine.

32. Exhale and place the palms facedown onto the tops of the thighs. If your bottom doesn't reach the floor, place a block or stack of books underneath for additional support.

33. Relax your shoulders by gently drawing the shoulder blades down the back and feel a gentle lift and softness through the neck and the eyes.

34. Stay in **Hero**, taking deep breaths for 30 seconds to a few minutes.

35. Release **Hero** and take a comfortable resting position for **Waves Visualization** (page 192).

INTERMEDIATE SEQUENCE 3

5 AND UP

 CALMING

 REJUVENATING

This is a great sequence to practice for stress or anxiety. A Body Scan: Short Version (page 184) sets the tone for this focused and rhythmic practice. The soothing rocking movements from Child's Pose (page 46) to Table Top (page 44) and Table Top to Down Dog (page 52) build a smooth and calming yoga practice. This sequence is great for connection and teamwork, as it also integrates partner poses.

1. **Body Scan: Short Version** (page 184).

2. Lie on your back for **Happy Baby** (page 92) and take a few rounds of breath.

3. Sit on the mat facing forward with your legs straight in front of you. Draw the right knee in toward your chest and place the right foot on the ground outside of your left thigh for **Seated Twist** (page 114).

4. To go deeper, on an exhale, take the left elbow outside the right knee and point your fingertips toward the ceiling.

5. Come back to center and draw the left knee in toward your chest and place the left foot on the ground outside your right thigh for **Seated Twist**, opposite side.

6. To go deeper, on an exhale, take the right elbow outside the left knee and point your fingertips toward the ceiling.

continued

7. Sit on a folded blanket, bolster or pillow. Shift your weight forward, bend your knees, and press the soles of your feet together for **Butterfly** (page 86). Rest your head in the arches of the feet, on top of the stacked fists, or cupped in your hands while the elbows rest on the feet. Breathe gently for approximately three minutes, **Yin Butterfly** (page 196).

8. Inhale as you come up, then stretch your legs forward and lean back on your hands. Relax for a few breaths here.

9. On an exhale, take **Child's Pose** (page 46), inhale to **Table Top** (page 44) and repeat this rhythmic movement with the breath three times.

10. From **Table Top**, breathe in, and on the exhale, press the hands down and the hips up and back to **Down Dog** (page 52). Repeat this motion three times.

11. Inhale in **Down Dog**, exhale into **Plank** (page 54).

12. From **Plank**, release down in a **Yoga Push-Up** (page 56) and lift the torso and upper body forward and up for **Up Dog** (page 120).

13. Press the hands down, and on an exhale, lift the hips to **Down Dog**.

14. Step the feet to the front of the mat, **Forward Fold** (page 42).

15. Inhale, press the feet down firmly, and lift the upper body up to **Mountain** (page 40).

16. Find a partner and set up for **Double Plank** (page 166). To release, Partner B steps the feet down and slowly lifts their hands off Partner A.

17. Step into **Mountain**, still facing each other.

18. Shift your weight into one leg and find a focal point for the eyes in front of you on the floor. Turn the other knee out toward the side of the room and lift the foot into **Tree** (page 134).

19. Mirror your **Tree** so Partner A is balancing on the right leg and Partner B is balancing on the left leg. Press your hands together at the top of your tree for **Double Tree** (page 156).

20. Repeat on the other side.

21. Step into **Mountain**, inhale.

22. Exhale, press the hands down to the mat, and step back to **Plank**.

23. Inhale, lower the knees for **Table Top**.

24. Sit back in **Criss-Cross** (page 100).

25. Face one another with your knees pulled in and up toward the ceiling and your feet on the floor. Move close enough to your partner so you can press your feet against hers. Begin to press the soles of the feet against one another, creating leverage and holding hands to build a deeper connection, **Double Boat** (page 164).

26. If straight knees are not possible, simply stay in the pose with the knees bent.

27. Take a few deep breaths and release the hands and feet to the ground.

28. Extend the legs in front of you and then bend the knees out-ward and draw the feet together with the soles of the feet touch-ing, **Butterfly**.

29. Sit up in **Criss-Cross** and turn back-to-back for **We Got This** breath (page 30). (If you have an odd number of people, try one group of three in a triangle with shoulders touching.) Take an inhale, and on the exhale say silently or aloud (depending on your mood) "We got this." Repeat three to five times.

INTERMEDIATE SEQUENCE 4

5 AND UP

 ENERGIZING

 STRENGTHENING

This sequence opens with a relaxing and soothing activity with Legs Up the Wall (page 190). Allow the mind to unwind first, then move into poses like Low Lunge Twist (page 116) and Twisting Triangle (page 118). You'll also engage the core with Boat pose (page 94) before you unwind it all again with Waves Visualization (page 192).

1. Place the yoga mat against a wall with plenty of clearance to lift the legs up. Have a folded blanket or two on hand to provide extra lift under the lower back for **Legs Up the Wall** (page 190). Stay here for a few minutes or longer, breathing gently and allowing gravity to relax the body.

2. Release the legs and lie on your back for **Happy Baby** (page 92) and take a few rounds of breath.

3. Draw your knees to your chest, rock back and forth a few times, and rock forward to **Table Top** (page 44).

4. Take a round of breath and exhale, **Down Dog** (page 52).

5. Step the right foot forward between the hands and set the left knee down for **Low Lunge** (page 76) right side.

6. Lift the torso and arms up, turn the body toward the right, and take the left hand to the outer right knee for **Low Lunge Twist** (page 116), right side. To go deeper, take the left elbow outside the right knee and press the palms together at the sternum.

7. Set the hands down on the mat, lift the hips, and press up and back to **Down Dog**.

8. Step the left foot between the hands and lower the right knee for **Low Lunge**, other side.

9. Lift the torso and arms up, turn the body toward the left, and take the right hand to the outer left knee for **Low Lunge Twist**, other side. To go deeper, take the right elbow outside the left knee and press the palms together at the sternum.

10. Release the twist and come back to a neutral position. Press the hands and knees down for **Table Top**.

11. Lift the hips up and back, **Down Dog**.

12. Inhale, step the right foot forward, and bend the front knee to a 90-degree angle for **Warrior 1** (page 66).

13. Extend the arms out and turn toward the side of the room, right knee still bent, for **Warrior 2** (page 68).

14. Place the right elbow on the top of the right thigh and reach the left arm up and over for **Side Angle** (page 78), right side.

15. Press firmly down into the feet, turn the left heel up toward the ceiling, and reach the arms overhead. Turn the torso toward the right, press the left hand into the right knee, and turn into **High Lunge Twist** (page 130), right side. To go deeper, take the left elbow outside the right knee and press the palms together at the sternum.

16. Press the hands down to the mat, and lift the hips up and back to **Down Dog**.

17. Step the left foot forward to the front of the mat, **Warrior 1**, left side.

18. Extend the arms open wide into **Warrior 2**, left side.

19. Place the left elbow on top of the left thigh for **Side Angle**, left side.

20. Press firmly down into the feet, turn the right heel up toward the ceiling, and reach the arms overhead. Turn the torso toward the left, press the right hand into the left knee, and turn into **High Lunge Twist**, left side. To go deeper, take the left elbow outside the right knee and press the palms together at the sternum.

continued

21. Inhale, press the hands down to the mat, and lift the hips up and back to **Down Dog**.

22. Exhale, press forward into **Plank** (page 54).

23. Inhale and exhale. From **Plank** release down in **Yoga Push-Up** (page 56) and inhale, lifting the torso and upper body forward and up for **Up Dog** (page 120).

24. On an exhale, press the hands down, and lift the hips up and back, **Down Dog**.

25. Step to the front of the mat, **Forward Fold** (page 42).

26. Press the feet down, lift the arms up and overhead into **Mountain** (page 40).

27. Step the left foot back for **Triangle** on the right side.

28. Press the feet down and turn into **Twisting Triangle** (page 118), right side. Turn your left foot in slightly as you reach both arms out to the side. Inhale deeply, draw the front hip slightly back, and reach the upper body forward. The back hip can move slightly forward to extend the upper body more. Rest the right hand on your shin, ankle, or the floor outside of your front foot.

Use a block or stack of books if this feels tight in the hamstrings. Reach the top arm straight up.

29. Press the feet down and lift the torso upright and take a breath. Now turn the torso to the right, shift the right hip back and reach your left arm forward. Take steady breaths as you turn the torso and twist from the core. Place the left hand outside the right foot or on an elevated prop, and reach the right arm directly above for **Twisting Triangle**, right side. To release, press the feet down, engage the core, and on an exhale, lift the torso back up.

30. Turn the body toward the left and turn the right and left foot so that both are facing the opposite side of the room from the Twisting Triangle. Take a deep breath and imagine you are getting longer through your spine. Lean the torso and arms forward toward the floor, using a block or stack of books to rest your hands on if the floor feels too far away. Allow your neck and shoulders to relax as you hinge forward for **Wide-Legged Forward Fold** (page 110).

31. Turn to the back of your mat and angle the right foot behind you; now the left foot is forward for **Triangle** on the left side.

32. Press the feet down and lift the torso upright and take a breath. Now turn the torso to the left, shift the left hip back, and reach the right arm forward. Take steady breaths as you turn the torso and twist from the core. Place the right arm outside the left foot or on an elevated prop, and reach the left arm directly above for **Twisting Triangle**, right side. To release, press the feet down, engage the core, and on an exhale, lift the torso back up.

33. Turn the body toward the right and turn the left and right foot so that both are facing the opposite side of the room from the Twisting Triangle. Take a deep breath and imagine your spine lengthening. Lean the torso and arms forward toward the floor, using a block or stack of books to rest your hands on if the floor feels too far away. Allow your neck and shoulders to relax as you hinge forward for **Wide-Legged Forward Fold**.

34. Release onto the ground in a seated position with the legs straight out in front of you. With the soles of the feet on the ground, bend the knees. Take the hands behind the knees to begin, engage the core muscles, and lift the feet off the ground so the calves and shins are parallel to the ground. Take a deep breath in and out. If you feel ready for more core engagement, release the hands from behind the knees and reach the arms straight out along your sides, palms facing one another. Relax your shoulders by gently drawing the shoulder blades down the back. It's your choice if you'd like to reach the legs straight up and away from you, forming a seated "V" shape with the body, **Boat** (page 94).

continued

35. Lie down on the mat. Keep your hands by the sides of the thighs, palms facing down. Bend your knees and draw your feet in toward your bottom. Inhale and relax the neck. Exhale and press the arms, hands, and feet down firmly, engage the core slightly, and raise the hips up with the thighs engaged and parallel to the ground. Lift the chin slightly and choose a spot on the ceiling to look at to build focus. Take a few deep breaths in **Bridge** (page 60).

36. Hug the knees toward your chest. Bend the knees and grab the outer edge of each foot with the respective hand: right hand grabs outer edge of right foot and left hand grabs outer edge of left foot. Allow the spine and lower back to release toward the ground, taking slow, deep breaths. If it feels comfortable and relaxing, you can rock from side to side holding the feet in **Happy Baby** (page 92).

37. Release **Happy Baby** and take a comfortable resting position for **Waves Visualization** (page 192).

ADVANCED SEQUENCE 1

7 AND UP

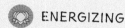 ENERGIZING

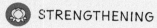 STRENGTHENING

The advanced sequence begins with active, rhythmic movements from Frog (page 82) to Mountain (page 40) and Forward Fold (page 42). Building momentum with fluid poses and breaths lets the body release anxiety and feel rejuvenated from the very start. As you build in this practice, you'll work on Handstand Variation (page 148), Boat (page 94), and deep relaxation with Legs Up the Wall (page 190).

1. Step your feet apart enough so that you can squat your bottom down toward the ground. Be liberal with the amount of space you give yourself. Take an inhale, and as you exhale, squat down toward the ground. If you need additional support for balance, try this against the wall. If you need additional height under the heels, you can roll up a couple of towels and place them underneath the heels. Press your palms together at your sternum and take a few deep breaths in **Frog** (page 82).

2. Release the hands and lift to **Mountain** (page 40).

3. Reach the arms up as you inhale, exhale, take a slight bend in the knees, and release down into **Forward Fold** (page 42).

4. Inhale, squat into **Frog**. Exhale.

5. Inhale, lift into **Mountain**.

6. Exhale, **Forward Fold**.

7. Inhale, **Frog**. Exhale.

8. Inhale, **Mountain**.

continued

9. Connect to your breath and keep it steady. Step your feet apart so that your feet are directly underneath your hips. Bend your knees and take your right knee over your left, squeeze the inner thighs together, and lower your bottom toward the ground, balancing on your left foot. If that feels unsteady, bend the left knee, squat down, and cross your right ankle over the left knee, making a modified "4" with the lower part of your body. Bring the arms forward, cross the arms with the right arm on top. Press the forearms and backs of the hands into each other, **Eagle** (page 136).

10. Stay connected to your breath. Bend your knees and take your left knee over your right, squeeze the inner thighs together, and lower your bottom toward the ground, balancing on your right foot. If that feels unsteady, bend the right knee, squat down, and cross your left ankle over the right knee, making a modified "4" with the lower part of your body. Bring the arms forward, cross the arms with the left arm on top. Press the forearms and backs of the hands into each other, **Eagle**.

11. Breathe and release into **Mountain**.

12. Exhale, **Forward Fold**. Inhale.

13. Exhale, press back into **Plank** (page 54), firm the hands, core, and thighs.

14. Inhale, lift the hips, **Down Dog** (page 52).

15. Exhale, **Plank**.

16. Inhale, **Down Dog**.

17. Exhale, **Plank**.

18. Inhale, **Down Dog**.

19. Exhale, **Plank**.

20. Inhale, lower the knees to the ground, **Table Top** (page 44).

21. Release onto the ground in a seated position with the legs straight out in front of you. Keeping the soles of the feet on the ground, bend the knees in. Take the hands behind the knees to begin, engage the core muscles, and lift the feet off the ground so the calves and shins are parallel to the ground. Take a deep breath in and out. If you feel ready for more core engagement, release the hands from behind the knees and reach the arms straight out along your sides, palms facing one another.

Relax your shoulders by gently drawing the shoulder blades down the back. Straighten the legs up and away from you, forming a seated "V" shape with the body. Breathe and focus in **Boat** (page 94) for at least five rounds of breath.

22. Set the feet down and shift forward into **Table Top**.

23. Reach the hands forward, extend the hips back, and elongate the spine as you take a few rounds of breath in **Puppy** (page 112).

24. Walk the hands back to **Table Top**, inhale, drop the belly, lift the chin, and gaze up toward the ceiling, **Cow** (page 50).

25. Exhale, curl the spine up toward the ceiling as you tuck the chin in toward the chest, **Cat** (page 48).

26. Inhale, **Cow**.

27. Exhale, **Cat**.

28. Inhale, **Cow**.

29. Exhale, **Cat**.

30. Inhale, **Table Top**.

31. Exhale, **Down Dog**.

32. Inhale, **Mountain**.

33. Exhale, lower into **Frog**.

34. Separate your thighs so they are slightly wider than your torso, but keep your feet as close together as possible. If your heels lift, use a block to stand on or even a folded towel or blanket. Reach your arms down to the ground and sneak the shoulders down toward the insides of the knees. Press the hands down into the ground firmly, feeling strength and stability through the entire arm. Find a spot in front of the hands to focus your gaze in **Crow** (page 146). Lift onto the balls of the feet and bend the elbows, pressing the shins against the back of the arms. Engage your core and practice lifting one foot off the ground. Keeping the core engaged, lift both feet off the ground, resting the knees against the backs of the arms as if they were on a little shelf. Use a few rounds of breath to stabilize the pose.

35. Exhale, jump or step the feet back from **Crow** to **Plank**. Inhale.

36. Exhale, **Down Dog**.

continued

37. Now place your yoga mat against a wall with plenty of space around you in all directions. Start in **Table Top** with the bottom of your feet pressing against the wall. Gradually walk the legs up the wall so that you are forming an "L" shape with your entire body. Keep the gaze just forward of your hands and breathe into the neck to soften it, even as the rest of the body is working hard. Make sure you have just the right amount of distance so that your shoulders are directly over the wrists. Press the hands firmly into the ground and press the right foot into the wall. Engage the core muscles and lift the left leg up straight toward the ceiling. If you feel steady, practice pressing the right foot into the wall even more for leverage and lift it up to meet the left leg, **Handstand Variation** (page 148).

38. Bring the legs down to the ground safely and move into **Down Dog** or **Child's Pose** (page 46).

39. Practice the pose again, lifting the right foot up first. Notice any difference in the pose or preference for sides.

40. Release the **Handstand Variation** and squat down for **Frog**. Keep your mat by the wall.

41. Reach the hands forward, extend the hips back, and elongate the spine as you take a few rounds of breath in **Puppy**.

42. Move to a modified **Candle** (page 74), standing on the knees directly under the hips, rather than on the feet. For added lift, tuck the toes under and lift the heels. For a deeper stretch, allow the tops of the feet to remain on the floor. Place your hands on your hips and then rotate the elbows so they point to the back of your mat behind you. The hands may rotate more to the back of the hips and pelvis now. Firm the shoulder blades onto the back and allow the hips to move forward slightly as you lift up and back through the torso and chest. The head and neck can relax backward as the chest lifts. If you feel steady and safe, you may reach the hands back and down to grab the heels. Relax your shoulders and neck by gently drawing the shoulder blades down the back, **Camel** (page 122). To release, engage through the core again, and take the hands back to the hips, lifting the body back up into modified **Candle** on the knees. The neck and head come up last.

43. Reach the hands forward, extend the hips back, and elongate the spine as you take a few rounds of breath in **Puppy**.

44. Release down and turn back toward the wall. Take your **Legs Up the Wall** (page 190) for three to five minutes.

ADVANCED SEQUENCE 2

7 AND UP

 ENERGIZING

 STRENGTHENING

This core-strengthening practice invites you to slow down. Breathing steadily while holding stationary poses can be quite challenging and invigorating. A series of warrior poses prepares the body for focus, followed by Standing Splits (page 128) and Side Plank (page 144). The key to this practice is the steady connection to your breath amid more challenging balances to build focus and confidence.

1. Press the hands and feet down into the ground with the hips elevated, and hold **Down Dog** (page 52) for five rounds of breath.

2. On an inhale, shift the hips back, firm the thighs, and engage the core for **Plank** (page 54), and hold for five rounds of breath.

3. On an exhale, extend back into **Down Dog**, and hold for seven rounds of breath.

4. Take a big inhale and exhale, move back into **Plank**, and hold for seven rounds of breath.

5. Release the knees down for **Table Top** (page 44) and one round of breath.

6. Exhale, **Down Dog**.

7. Inhale, step forward into **Mountain** (page 40).

8. Step the left foot back, bend the right knee to a 90-degree angle, and turn the left foot out to a 45-degree angle, simultaneously angling the hips slightly forward. Press the feet into the ground firmly. Take a deep breath in and lift both arms above the head, **Warrior 1** (page 66). Inhale.

9. Exhale, extend the arms wide to either side, turn the torso toward the left, and reach into **Warrior 2** (page 68). Take a round of breath here.

10. Exhale, press into the left toes and ball of the foot as you turn the heel up toward the ceiling. Breathe in and lean your weight forward into the right foot as you lift the left foot and left leg into the air, parallel to the ground like an airplane. Take a deep breath and reach the arms forward, palms facing each other, as the leg lifts and the back foot presses back as if into a wall. Find your focal point on the ground. Spend a few rounds of breath here in **Warrior 3** (page 140), building focus and stability.

11. Inhale and exhale, release the hands toward the floor or the right ankle as you lift the left leg firmly into the air for **Standing Splits** (page 128). Take a few rounds of breath here.

12. On an exhale, set the left foot down next to the right, **Forward Fold** (page 42).

13. Inhale, lift the torso and reach the arms up, **Mountain**.

14. Step the right foot back, bend the left knee to a 90-degree angle and turn the right foot out to a 45-degree, simultaneously angling the hips slightly forward. Press the feet into the ground firmly. Take a deep breath in and lift both arms above the head, **Warrior 1**. Inhale.

15. Exhale, extend the arms wide to either side, turn the torso toward the right, and reach into **Warrior 2**. Take a round of breath here.

16. Exhale, press into the right toes and ball of the foot as you turn the heel up toward the ceiling. Breathe in and lean your weight forward into the left foot as you lift the right foot and right leg into the air, parallel to the ground like an airplane. Take a deep breath and reach the arms forward, palms facing each other, as the leg lifts and the back foot presses back as if into a wall. Find your focal point on the ground. Spend a few rounds of breath here in **Warrior 3**, building focus and stability.

continued

17. Inhale and exhale, release the hands toward the floor or the left ankle as you lift the right leg firmly into the air for **Standing Splits**. Take a few rounds of breath here.

18. Release the right leg next to the left, **Forward Fold**.

19. Step the left foot back, **High Lunge** (page 80). Set your left hand down near the inside of the right foot. Breathe in and lengthen the right arm directly up, then breathe out. Breathe deeply again and lengthen the spine, twisting toward the right a bit more. Relax your shoulders by gently drawing the shoulder blades down the back, **High Lunge Twist** (page 130).

20. On an exhale, press the hands down and lift the hips up and back, **Down Dog**. Inhale.

21. Exhale, **Plank**.

22. Stay in **Plank**, take a deep inhale, and shift the weight onto the right hand, rolling onto the outer edge of the right foot. Press the feet together, reach the left arm up, making a straight line with the right arm, engage your core muscles, and press the hand into the ground firmly. Take a deep breath and hold your gaze steady toward the side of the room for **Side Plank** (page 144). While the arms and legs work to engage the pose, relax the eyes and neck. Hold steady for a few rounds of breath.

23. On an exhale, release back into **Plank**.

24. Inhale, move the torso and chest forward and up as the thighs lift off the ground, **Up Dog** (page 120).

25. Exhale, **Down Dog**.

26. Inhale, step the feet to the front of the mat, **Forward Fold**. Exhale.

27. Inhale, **Mountain**.

28. Exhale, step the right foot back, **High Lunge**. Set your right hand down near the inside of the left foot. Breathe in and lengthen the left arm directly up, then breathe out. Breathe deeply again and lengthen the spine, twisting toward the left a bit more. Relax your shoulders by gently drawing the shoulder blades down the back, **High Lunge Twist**.

29. On an exhale, press the hands down, and lift the hips up and back, **Down Dog**. Inhale.

30. Exhale, **Plank**.

31. Stay in **Plank**, take a deep inhale, and shift the weight onto the left hand, rolling onto the outer edge of the left foot. Press the feet together, reach the right arm up, making a straight line with the left arm, engage your core muscles, and press the hand into the ground firmly. Take a deep breath and hold your gaze steady toward the side of the room for **Side Plank**. While the arms and legs work to engage the pose, relax the eyes and neck. Hold steady for a few rounds of breath.

32. Exhale, **Plank**.

33. Inhale, move the torso and chest forward and up as the thighs lift off the ground, **Up Dog**.

34. Exhale, **Down Dog**. Take a few rounds of breath here.

35. Exhale, knees down for **Table Top**.

36. Inhale, then exhale and extend forward for **Puppy** (page 112).

37. Lie face down on the floor with your belly and tops of the feet on the ground. Draw the feet in toward your bottom closely. Lift the torso and chest as you reach back with your hands to the outer edges of the feet for **Bow** (page 126). Even as you lift and stretch back to hold the feet, allow the belly to feel softer and relax your eyes. Relax your shoulders by gently drawing the shoulder blades down the back. Release the legs and gently lower the upper body and legs to the floor.

38. Roll onto your back. Hug the knees toward your chest. Bend the knees and grab the outer edge of each foot with the respective hand: right hand grabs outer edge of right foot and left hand grabs outer edge of left foot. Allow the spine and lower back to release toward the ground, taking slow, deep breaths. If it feels comfortable and relaxing, you can rock from side to side holding the feet in **Happy Baby** (page 92).

39. Release **Happy Baby** and take a comfortable resting position for **Body Scan: Long Version** (page 186).

CHAPTER

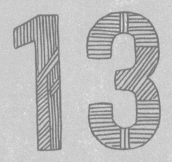

MEDITATIONS

Meditation is a practice of building awareness through focus on a single idea, physical sensation, or physical object. Meditation has been proven to change the development of the brain, increasing neural pathways that help us build concentration and creativity. Encouraging your little one to meditate can be daunting at first. As with any activity in this book, use your own sense of conviction and make it as fun as possible. When meditation becomes a routine, there are many rewards, including a sense of calm, serenity, reduced anxiety and depression, and improved focus. Encourage kids to notice how they feel both before and after meditation. Don't be discouraged if the results are initially negative. When we slow down, we come into closer contact with how we truly feel, and uncomfortable sensations like sadness or anger may arise. It's helpful to explain to children that it can be a challenge to sit still. Explain that your mind wanders also, and sometimes you don't feel like meditating in the beginning.

When practicing these meditations initially, the grown-up should take the role of the narrator, guiding children with the script and helping everyone ease into the meditation practice.

CONCENTRATION MEDITATION

ALL AGES

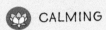 CALMING

Building concentration is an incredibly soothing and powerful practice. This meditation asks us to simply pay attention to the inhale and exhale. What is not always so simple is quieting the running inventory in our minds: to-do lists, worries, fears, excitement, and planning all consume storage space up there. When we practice concentrating on the breath, we can begin to remove some of the mental clutter, even if temporarily. For younger children, try reducing the time even to 10 seconds and narrate what's happening more in the beginning. Build up from there. On the flip side, if 3 minutes seems achievable and easy, increase the amount of time you meditate up to 10 minutes or longer.

1. Find a position that's comfortable for you. You can sit Criss-Cross (page 100) on your yoga mat or in a chair, or even lie on the ground. The important thing is to find a position where you can feel relaxed and keep fidgeting to a minimum.

2. Close your eyes or keep the gaze soft and inward-facing (try not to dart the eyes around the room).

3. Elongate through the spine in whatever position you've chosen. As the spine elongates, relax the neck and shoulders. Take one deep inhale through the nose, and open the mouth to exhale with an "ahhh" sound.

4. Imagine that you can breathe directly into the belly, and relax all the muscles there.

5. Set a timer for three minutes or less with a sound that is soothing and calming for you.

6. Notice the quality of your breathing: Is it shallow? Quick? Steady? Even? Allow your attention to your breathing to feel as gentle and soothing as possible. Find comfort in the rhythm of the inhale and the exhale.

7. Keep your attention on your breath without trying to control the quality of your breathing. Unlike yoga practice or breathing practice, we're no longer trying to take deep breaths.

8. Continue to simply bring your attention back to your breathing. When your mind wanders, guide it gently back to focus on your breath.

9. When the timer goes off, open your eyes gently and notice how you feel.

CANDLE MEDITATION

ALL AGES

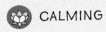 CALMING

This is a concentration meditation that takes the focus away from our breath and places it on an object. It's best to use a flameless LED flicker light for safety purposes. You can also use any other soothing object to focus the eyes. This meditation almost tricks the brain into slowing down thoughts and feelings. When we focus and concentrate on something external, it automatically takes our attention away from the chatter of the mind. This means you are unable to worry, anticipate, remember, or hook into other common distractions while meditating on the candle. Kids may find this easier than the simple Concentration Meditation (page 234), since it involves something to look at and watch.

1. Start in Criss-Cross (page 100).

2. Keep your eyes open and allow them to gently focus on the candle. Keep the gaze soft and inward facing (try not to dart the eyes around the room).

3. Sit up nice and tall. As the spine elongates, relax the neck and shoulders. Take one deep inhale through the nose, and open the mouth to exhale with an "ahhh" sound.

4. Imagine you can breathe directly into the belly, and relax all the muscles there.

5. Set a timer for 3 to 10 minutes with a sound that is soothing and calming for you.

6. Keep your focus on the candle and do not allow it to stray elsewhere.

7. Notice when you feel an impulse to look somewhere else and continue to hold the gaze steady on the candle.

8. You can give yourself simple (and silent) words of encouragement like "Wow. You really want to look around the room. It's okay. You've got this. Just a few more minutes."

9. Continue to simply bring your attention back to the candle. When your mind wanders, guide it gently back to focus on the candle.

10. When the timer goes off, gently bring your attention back to the room, and notice how you feel.

COMPASSION MEDITATION

5 AND UP

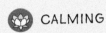 CALMING

Uncover feelings of kindness and love during this meditation. Using our imagination here, we think of someone we love and how that person makes us feel. When we imagine someone who loves us unconditionally, we can actually sense the feeling of love, which provides comfort through difficult times even if that person isn't physically with us. And when we imagine the love we feel for another, we are reminded of the strong connections we have with our family and friends. This is a great practice for times of loneliness or hurt feelings and an opportunity to teach kids about the power of unconditional love.

1. Start in Criss-Cross (page 100).

2. Close your eyes or keep the gaze soft and inward-facing (try not to dart the eyes around the room).

3. Sit up nice and tall. As the spine elongates, relax the neck and shoulders. Take one deep inhale through the nose, and open the mouth to exhale with an "ahhh" sound.

4. Imagine you can breathe directly into your belly, and relax all the muscles there.

5. Set a timer for 3 to 10 minutes with a sound that is soothing and calming for you.

6. Imagine someone you love (this can also be a pet), who fills your heart with warmth, and pretend you can see that person or being in front of you.

7. Connect to your inhale and exhale.

8. Imagine you have a beautiful golden light in your heart, like sunlight. You have the magical power to send this light out to the person in front of you.

9. Breathing in and out, feel the light in your heart expand and glow even stronger toward the person in front of you.

10. You can silently say to the image of your loved one in front of you "May you be happy. May you be free."

11. Now release the image of the person, but keep feeling that warm, golden light in your heart.

12. Focus your attention on yourself and your heart. Say silently to yourself "May I be happy. May I be free."

13. Take a few more rounds of breath, and connect to that warm glow inside your heart.

14. Open your eyes gently and notice how you feel.

GRATITUDE MEDITATION

3 AND UP

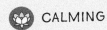 CALMING

Expressing gratitude and appreciation is linked to greater happiness. Use this meditation as an opportunity to feel grateful for each other and all the gifts in your life. Gratitude is a way to simply celebrate all that helps us move through life, for example health, family, home, friends, pets, nature, and more. When we choose to be still, connect to our breath, and take a few moments (or longer) to truly appreciate all that we have, we build a stronger sense of optimism and connection. Remembering our gifts is a way to connect to our innate sense of peace and compassion. Kids are particularly good at gratitude—let them inspire you! As you sit together in the Gratitude Meditation, allow the busyness of everyday life to wash away, and connect to what truly matters for you and your family.

1. Start in Criss-Cross (page 100).

2. Close your eyes or keep the gaze soft and inward-facing (try not to dart the eyes around the room).

3. Sit up nice and tall. As the spine elongates, relax the neck and shoulders. Take one deep inhale through the nose, and open the mouth to exhale with an "ahhh" sound.

4. Imagine you can breathe directly into your belly, and relax all the muscles there.

5. Set a timer for 3 to 10 minutes with a sound that is soothing and calming for you.

6. Connect to your inhale and exhale.

7. As you breathe, connect with the small and large gifts in your life: the people, places, and things that help sustain you.

8. Breathe in and out, and feel grateful for the everyday gift of surrounding nature.

9. Breathe in and out, and feel grateful for family and friends.

10. **Breathe in and out, and express gratitude for your health.**

11. **Breathe in and out, and feel gratitude toward yourself for all your efforts every day and for all the unique assets you bring to the world.**

12. **Take a few more silent moments, allowing any other spontaneous ideas about gratitude to arise and fill your heart with appreciation.**

13. **Open your eyes gently and notice how you feel.**

WALKING MEDITATION

3 AND UP

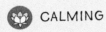 CALMING

Walking meditation is a wonderful way to integrate movement into the practice of meditation and can be a great starting place if you have a little one who struggles to sit still. This meditation still requires a great amount of concentration, but the slow movement can help channel excess energy. Walking Meditation can be done in a public park, more remote in nature, the backyard, or anywhere where you have room to take 10 steps. Walking slowly might look or feel funny at first, but stick with it! Notice how moving slowly invites you to build a mind-body connection. If you or your child accidentally speed up, come back to the present moment by simply saying "Just here, just now" and continuing with your slow steps. Absorb the sights and sounds around you as you walk and meditate.

1. Find an inviting place to take at least 10 steps forward and back.

2. To start, stand still and feel your feet on the ground.

3. Imagine you can breathe directly into your belly, and relax all the muscles there.

4. Take a slow, deliberate step and notice the feeling of the foot lifting off the ground. Notice the sights and sounds around you.

5. Continue to take slow, deliberate steps and count them, ultimately walking forward 10 steps.

6. As you walk, connect to your inhale and exhale, and continue to be aware of the sights and sounds surrounding you, maintaining a steadiness with your gaze.

7. Continue to notice how your legs and arms feel as you walk.

8. Connect to your inhale and exhale, and when you have taken 10 steps, turn around to take 10 more steps back, toward your starting place if possible.

9. When complete, notice how you feel. Did slowing down your movements and connecting to your breath create any new feelings or sensations?

SLEEPYTIME MEDITATION

ALL AGES

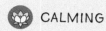 CALMING

Who doesn't a want to unwind and relax before bedtime? This is important for kids and adults alike. Stick with this one if your child resists at first; learning how to care for your body and mind prior to sleep has profound lasting benefits. A simple practice of belly breathing connects us to the rhythm and pace of the breath as it slows down. You may even find yourself or your little one drifting off to sleep mid-practice, a wonderful conclusion!

1. Start in bed, relaxed and ready for a good night's sleep. Close your eyes.

2. Take one deep inhale through the nose, and open the mouth to exhale with an "ahhh" sound.

3. Imagine you can breathe directly into your belly, and relax all the muscles there.

4. Relax the muscles in the shoulders, neck, jaw, and all the surrounding areas.

5. Take your hands to your belly and fill your belly up like a balloon as you inhale. Exhale, and feel the belly relax back and down toward the bed.

6. Take a few more Balloon Breaths (page 29) in and out, relaxing more and more with each exhale.

7. Now imagine a balloon above you, and as you inhale, fill it with your entire day; anything that is worrying you or even all the fun you had. Exhale, and imagine the balloon drifting off as your eyes get heavier and your whole body feels more relaxed.

8. Allow this meditation to conclude naturally if everyone is sleepy, or after a few minutes simply turn off the lights.

"I AM" MEDITATION

ALL AGES

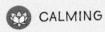 CALMING

Similar to the "I Am" Breath (page 34), the meditative repetition of soothing words here has the power to transform and calm. It's important to note that using an affirmative statement is not meant to deny any feelings that may be perceived as negative, like anger, sadness, or fear. When using an "I Am" Meditation, we can acknowledge challenging feelings first as we close our eyes and connect inside. The point of this meditation is to remind us that we are complex and carry peace inside us at all times. Try it out and witness the power of tapping into a sense of calm and peace within, even as other strong feelings call for your attention.

1. Find a position that's comfortable for you. You can sit Criss-Cross (page 100) on your yoga mat or in a chair, or lie on the ground. The important thing is to find a position where you can feel relaxed and keep fidgeting to a minimum.

2. Close your eyes or keep the gaze soft and inward-facing (try not to dart the eyes around the room).

3. Sit up nice and tall and elongate through the spine in whatever position you've chosen. As the spine elongates, relax the neck and shoulders. Take one deep inhale in through the nose, and open the mouth to exhale with an "ahhh" sound.

4. Imagine you can breathe directly into your belly, and relax all the muscles there.

5. Set a timer for 3 to 10 minutes with a sound that is soothing and calming for you.

6. Choose a quality to cultivate in your life—some examples include love, peace, calm, and strength. As you breathe in say to yourself "I am" and as you breathe out say the particular quality you want to cultivate. For the purposes of this example, we will use "Peace."

7. Inhale, "I am," exhale, "Peace."

8. Repeat "I am" on the inhale and "Peace" on the exhale for several rounds.

9. Continue to simply bring your attention back to your breathing and your "I am" statement.

10. Continue for as long as this feels soothing and helpful.

11. When the timer goes off, gently open your eyes and notice how you feel.

COUNTING MEDITATION

ALL AGES

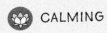 CALMING

Counting numbers may sound simple, but this practice holds tremendous power to build concentration, focus, and soothe the nervous system. When we are focused on counting, we cannot engage with any of the other busyness in the mind like planning, remembering, or worrying.

The discipline required to connect to our breath and count provides an even and steady focus for the mind. An active mind is channeled during a counting meditation. A great introduction to meditation, this meditation can also be integrated on the fly. Close your eyes and take three deep breaths three times a day and see what happens. Sometimes the simplest practices have the most profound effect.

1. Find a position that's comfortable for you. You can sit Criss-Cross (page 100) on your yoga mat or in a chair, or even lie on the ground. The important thing is to find a position where you can feel relaxed and keep fidgeting to a minimum.

2. Close your eyes or keep the gaze soft and inward-facing (try not to dart the eyes around the room).

3. Sit up nice and tall and elongate through the spine in whatever position you've chosen. As the spine elongates, relax the neck and shoulders. Take one deep inhale in through the nose, and open the mouth to exhale with an "ahhh" sound.

4. Imagine you can breathe directly into your belly, and relax all the muscles there.

5. Set a timer for 3 to 10 minutes with a sound that is soothing and calming for you.

6. Allow the breath to be fluid and natural (uncontrolled), and begin counting backward from 20.

7. Pause in between each number and allow the mind to focus solely on counting backward.

8. If you lose track of the numbers, simply start over.

9. If you find this practice to be soothing and the timer has not gone off, choose another number and begin counting backward again.

10. When the timer goes off, gently open your eyes and notice how you feel.

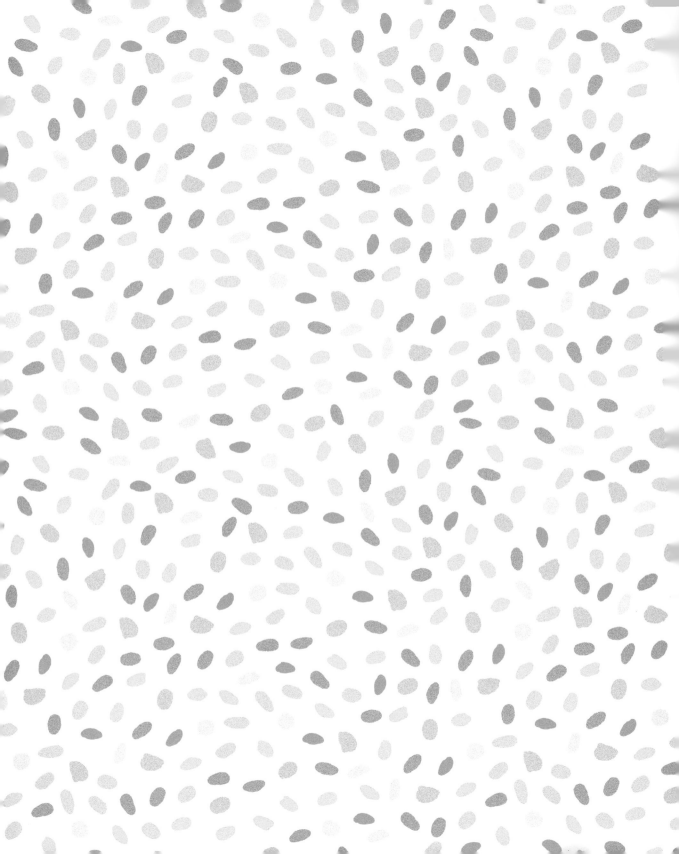

In Closing

YOGA HAS THE POWER TO TRANSFORM OUR LIVES. Whether you practice for five minutes or five hours (some people do!), the power of a deep breath is just as important as the power of Down Dog. Unplugging and spending time together in a healthy and nurturing way models self-care for our children.

Some of the best "yoga moments" I've had with my daughters have been spontaneous and fun. Olive, the oldest, has taken it upon herself to jump from Star into Mountain and back again a few times whenever she walks over a crack in the sidewalk. This makes for a long walk but gives her a feeling of ownership and joy—and as her mother, I can't argue with that!

Allow the poses and exercises in this book to sink in and integrate over time. Now that you've gained some experience, be open to how the yoga practices take shape for you and your youngsters. Yoga truly is a lifelong practice. Life evolves and so do we as individuals, as families, and collectively in our greater communities. Give yourself space to allow your yoga practice to grow.

The natural ebb and flow of life causes our tastes and preferences to change. If, for example, you (or your child) once loved doing partner poses but now they feel like a chore, practice acceptance and focus your sessions on other activities instead. On the flip side, give yourself permission to enjoy aspects of yoga that were once challenging. In my beginner yoga days, I *loathed* Triangle pose. I remember a teacher telling me to "feel my legs and feet grounding down," and I did an internal eye roll because I had no idea what she was talking about. Of course, I tried my best. I practiced hundreds of Triangle poses, struggling and confused, until years later it became one of my favorite poses. The key words here are *years later*—so take your time with yoga and go with the flow.

Ultimately, family yoga time is a time for connection and self-care. You get to choose the tone and approach that work best for your family. Enjoy digging into life's twists and turns with the great resource of yoga and the reliable tools of mindfulness. The individual and universal benefits are profound.

Yoga Library

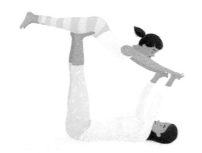

AIRPLANE, 160–161

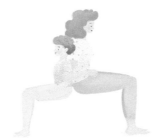

BACK-TO-BACK CHAIR, 154–155

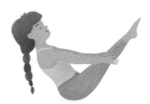

BOAT, 94–95

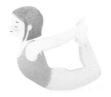

BOW, 126–127

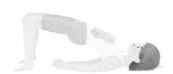

BRIDGE, 60–61

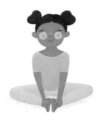

BUTTERFLY, 86–87

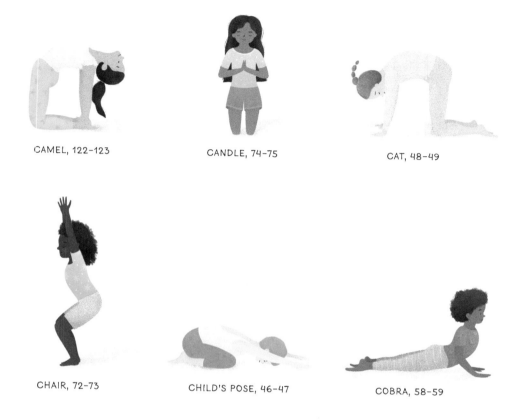

CAMEL, 122–123

CANDLE, 74–75

CAT, 48–49

CHAIR, 72–73

CHILD'S POSE, 46–47

COBRA, 58–59

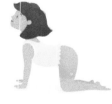

COW, 50–51

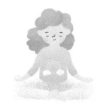

CRISS-CROSS, 100–101

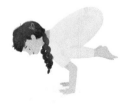

CROW, 146–147

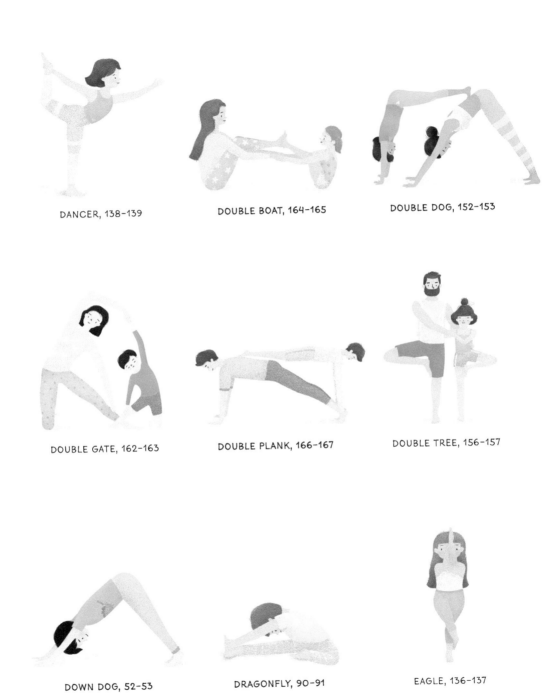

DANCER, 138–139

DOUBLE BOAT, 164–165

DOUBLE DOG, 152–153

DOUBLE GATE, 162–163

DOUBLE PLANK, 166–167

DOUBLE TREE, 156–157

DOWN DOG, 52–53

DRAGONFLY, 90–91

EAGLE, 136–137

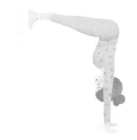

FORWARD FOLD, 42–43

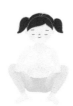

FROG, 82–83

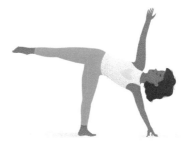

HALF MOON, 142–143

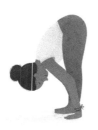

HANDSTAND VARIATION, 148–149

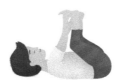

HAPPY BABY, 92–93

HERO, 96–97

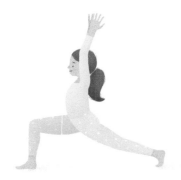

HIGH LUNGE, 80–81

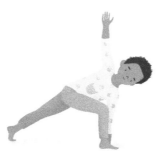

HIGH LUNGE TWIST, 130–131

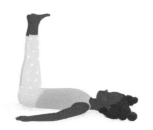

LEGS UP THE WALL, 190–191

YOGA LIBRARY

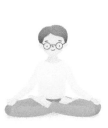

LOTUS, 102–103

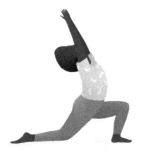

LOW LUNGE, 76–77

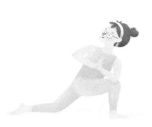

LOW LUNGE TWIST, 116–117

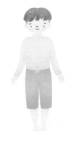

MOUNTAIN, 40–41

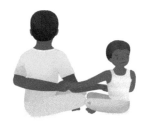

PARTNER SEATED TWIST, 158–159

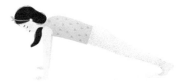

PLANK, 54–55

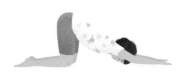

PUPPY, 112–113

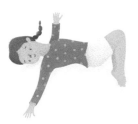

RECLINED TWIST, 108–109

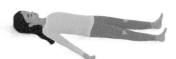

REST POSE, 182–183

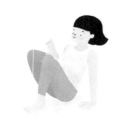

SEATED FIGURE "4", 104–105

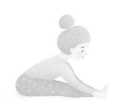

SEATED FORWARD BEND, 88–89

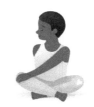

SEATED TWIST, 114–115

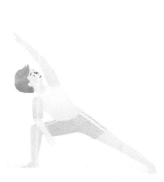

SIDE ANGLE, 78–79

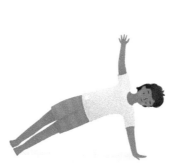

SIDE PLANK, 144–145

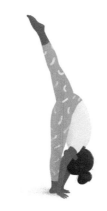

STANDING SPLITS, 128–129

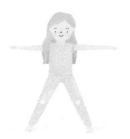

STAR, 64–65

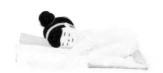

SUPPORTED CHILD'S POSE, 194–195

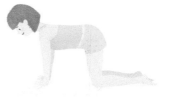

TABLE TOP, 44–45

YOGA LIBRARY

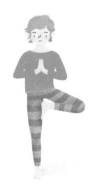

TREE, 134–135

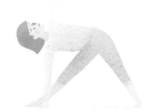

TRIANGLE, 70–71

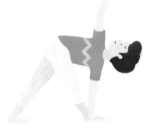

TWISTING TRIANGLE, 118–119

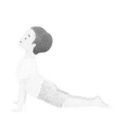

UP DOG, 120–121

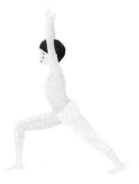

WARRIOR 1, 66–67

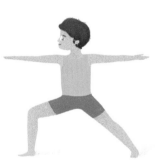

WARRIOR 2, 68–69

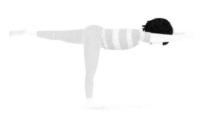

WARRIOR 3, 140–141

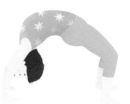

WHEEL, 124–125

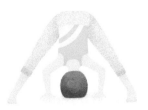

WIDE-LEGGED FORWARD
FOLD, 110–111

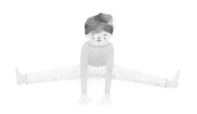

WIDE-LEGGED SEATED
FORWARD BEND, 98–99

YIN BUTTERFLY, 196–197

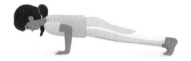

YOGA PUSH-UP, 56–57

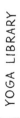

Resources

Headstand (Headstand.org)
A nonprofit dedicated to the integration of yoga and mindfulness in K–12 schools.

Time In Kid (TimeInKid.com)
The creative mindfulness resource for modern parents with mindful attitudes.

Yoga Journal (YogaJournal.com)
The online resource for information regarding yoga poses, sequences, and editorial content.

Little Flower Yoga (LittleFlowerYoga.com)
A resource for kids' yoga poses.

***Light on Yoga* by B. K. S. Iyengar**
The quintessential yoga book to deepen your knowledge about yoga poses and philosophy.

***Insight Yoga* by Sarah Powers**
A beautifully photographed book with yoga philosophy and a guide to yin yoga.

Yogaland Podcast (Acast.com/yogaland)
A yoga podcast by the journalist Andrea Ferretti.

***Yoga for Children* by Lisa Flynn**
A yoga-for-kids resource book.

Spirit Rock (SpiritRock.org)
A West Coast think tank for meditation and mindfulness with retreats and other offerings.

Kripalu (Kripalu.org)
An East Coast yoga retreat center.

OM Schooled (OM-Schooled.com)
Kids' yoga training and writing by the multitalented Sarah Herrington.

YogaGlo (YogaGlo.com)
The premiere online yoga studio.

Cosmic Kids (CosmicKids.com)
Playful yoga videos for younger children.

mindful (mindful.org)
The online resource for meditation and mindfulness.

Pacific Pause (PacificPause.com)
A meditation blog and studio by mom and former corporate executive and private equity guru Jing Cai Lee.

References

Anders, Mark. "Does Yoga Really Do the Body Good?" *ACE Fitness Matters*.
September/October 2005. https://www.acefitness.org/getfit/studies
/YogaStudy2005.pdf

Centers for Disease Control and Prevention and the Health Resources and Services
Administration. Key Findings: "Trends in the Parent-Report of Health Care
Provider-Diagnosed and Medicated ADHD: United States, 2003–2011."
https://www.cdc.gov/ncbddd/adhd/features/key-findings-adhd72013.html

Hözel, Britta K., James Carmody, Mark Vangel, Christina Congleton, Sita M.
Yerramsetti, Tim Gard, Sara W. Lazar. "Mindfulness practice leads to increases
in regional brain matter density." *Psychiatry Research: Neuroimaging*. 191,
no. 1 (30 January 2011): 36–43.

M. Jay Polsgrove, Brandon M. Eggleston, and Roch J. Lockyer. "Impact of 10-weeks
of Yoga Practice on Flexibility and Balance of College Athletes." *International
Journal of Yoga* 9, no. 1 (January–June 2016): 27–34. https://www.ncbi.nlm.nih.gov
/pmc/articles/PMC4728955/

Mindful. "John Kabat-Zinn: Defining Mindfulness." *Elephant* (January 11, 2017).
https://www.mindful.org/jon-kabat-zinn-defining-mindfulness.

"Yoga for Anxiety and Depression." *Harvard Health Publishing*. Harvard University.
Last modified September 18, 2017. https://www.health.harvard.edu
/mind-and-mood/yoga-for-anxiety-and-depression

Index of Yoga Activities

Index

About the Author

Katherine Priore Ghannam is the founder of Headstand, a nonprofit organization based in the San Francisco Bay Area. Leading a national movement to integrate mindfulness and yoga in K–12 schools, she oversees school programming, fundraising, strategic partnerships, and organizational sustainability. Katherine leads workshops training teachers around the country and strategizes with school leaders to develop cultural shifts for greater wellness in K–12 schools. She began her studies in mindfulness and yoga 17 years ago as a way to relieve stress as a public school teacher. Katherine is the recipient of a Jefferson Award for outstanding service to her community and has been featured on CBS and NBC news for her commitment to building more serene and sustainable environments for K–12 students and teachers. Katherine's new app, Time In Kid, is the creative mindfulness resource for kids and parents who want to spend time in, not time out.

CPSIA information can be obtained
at www.ICGtesting.com
Printed in the USA
LVHW010143231119
638193LV00001B/1

9 781939 754899